Ovarian Cyst Treatment

Dr. Steven Vasilev MD

DISCOVER ALL YOUR OPTIONS

America's Integrative Minimally Invasive Ovarian Surgeon

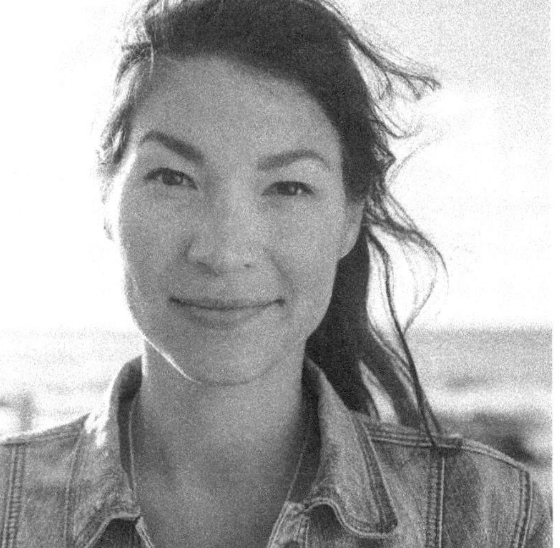

A Gift For My Readers

Visit OvaryDoctor.com to get your invitation to join Dr. Steven Vasilev MD for a free and informative online WEBINAR which digs deeper into ovarian cyst treatment from A to Z.

www.OvaryDoctor.com

Dr. Steven A. Vasilev MD MBA FACOG FACS FACN ABIHM ABOIM

America's first and leading quadruple board certified integrative gynecologic oncologist who specializes in advanced minimally invasive robotic surgery.

Clinical Professor, Loma Linda University School of Medicine

Medical Director & Professor, Integrative Gynecologic Oncology
Providence Saint John's Health Center and John Wayne Cancer Institute

Founding Director, Gynecologic Oncology Institute
(www.GynecologicOncologyInstitute.org)

Also by
Dr. Steven A. Vasilev MD

Cancer Cureology:
The Ultimate Survivor's Holistic Guide:
Integrative, Natural, Anti-Cancer Answers:
The Science And Truth

Gynecologic Oncology:
Evidence-Based Perioperative and Supportive Care

Coming Soon To Your Favorite Bookstores:
How Not To Get Cancer AGAIN

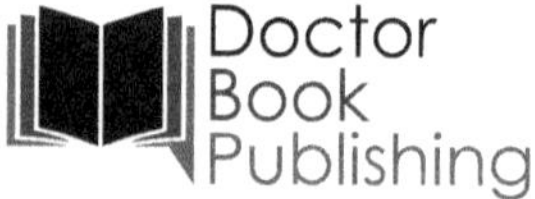

Published by:
Doctor Book Publishing
1775 Eye Street, NW
Suite 1150
Washington, DC 20006
1-800-704-3447

Ovarian Cyst Treatment

ISBN-13: 978-1-942065-27-2

Important Disclaimer: The author of this book, in collaboration with a fact-checking research team, is a quadruple board certified cancer surgeon who has been treating women with ovarian cysts over the past 35 years. This message is here to STRONGLY emphasize that this book and/or any information posted on my websites related to ovarian cysts are provided for INFORMATIONAL PURPOSES ONLY. Everyone is different and every situation is different which requires personal attention from a trusted and licensed health care provider in your area. None of the information herein is a substitute for professional medical advice, examination, diagnosis, or treatment. Always seek the advice of a physician or other qualified healthcare provider with any questions you may have regarding a medical condition or anything you read in this or any other book or website. Never disregard professional medical advice, or delay seeking it, because of something you have read in reports or books such as this or on websites. If you think you may have a medical emergency, call your doctor, 911 or your local emergency service immediately.

Any statements regarding herbal and supplement support in this book have not been evaluated by the *Food and Drug Administration*, according to which these products are not intended to diagnose, treat, cure or prevent any disease.

This book is dedicated to women of all ages battling ovarian cysts, endometriosis and ovarian cancer worldwide. Arm yourself with the information contained within and seek an early correct diagnosis to save a lot of pain and suffering.

Table of Contents

Introduction
VERY IMPORTANT

Many readers often skip the introduction in a book. PLEASE do not do that with this one. This is critical background information without which you won't understand where this book is coming from and how it can help save you a lot of pain!

So, first of all, what are ovarian cysts, how did they get there, are they all the same kind and are you sure you have an ovarian cyst? *If you did not ask these* ***four questions****, you may be on the* ***wrong path*** *towards getting rid of the type of ovarian cyst, or other ovary-related problem that you have.* Without knowing the answer you may be heading for unnecessary treatment, including surgery. On the other hand, you may be avoiding surgery that you really need. If someone tried to treat you without explaining the differences, you may be working with the wrong health practitioner, no matter if they are a gynecologist, surgeon, allopath, naturopath or homeopath.

Don't worry. You're not alone in having any of these cysts, but there are DEFINITELY more than a few different kinds. Literally millions of women have various types of cysts grow on their ovaries during their lifetime, sometimes once but usually many times. The key to successful treatment and prevention is to realize that there is no "one-size-fits-all" type of "cure", whether someone is hawking a top-secret cure or otherwise. That would be like saying that the best gas for your car is *also* very good for washing the car or putting into your cooling system. For the best chance of a "cure" you have to look for what will work for the type of problem and specific ovarian cyst or mass YOU have! You probably look for specific answers to specific problems and questions in all other parts of your life, right? This is no different, and is even more important. Your health hangs in the balance.

In order to help with the reducing symptoms of cysts, while you are working on eliminating them, you need to know WHY you are having the symptoms you are having. Otherwise, for example, it's sort of like trying to treat frostbite with ice packs because ice packs are good to treat other types of injury. Doesn't make sense does it? Ice packs might be good for treating various types of sprains for example, but that does not mean they are good for every kind of pain or injury. It is quite a bit more complicated than that with ovarian cyst symptoms, but the answers are laid out for you in this book.

It's critical to understand that most ovarian cysts can be successfully treated medically and naturally, but ovarian *tumors* can't. Both can look like cystic masses on ultrasound or they can feel the same when a doctor examines your pelvis. Tumors can be benign or malignant, but they NEVER go away on their own and can threaten your life. This is a crucial distinction that you need to find the answer to before wasting time or putting off a surgery that you might really need. In some cases, that surgery can save your life. On the other hand, you need to know enough to avoid a surgery you may NOT need. *You are about to discover how to find out everything you need to know to make the right choice for YOU!*

By the way, my strong advice to you is to maintain some healthy skepticism about anything you read. What is included in this book is based on reliable published resources, some of which I provided for you at the end of this book. You deserve to know if the evidence for any given recommendation is GREAT, or so-so, or completely bogus, unclear or unproven. It's up to you what you do with that information. At the end of the day, it's your body and your choice. But you still deserve to know. The research included in this book includes materials from the USA, Europe, China, India…essentially from the whole world…including mainstream and alternative thoughts from all of these regions on our planet.

First Things First: Anatomy and Physiology

HOW YOUR REPRODUCTIVE ORGANS LOOK AND WORK

Before talking about "cures" or treatments of any kind, it's critical to review how things look and work normally. So, the first thing we need to do is to review the basic anatomy and physiology of the ovaries, Fallopian (uterine) tubes, and uterus. These are your main gynecologic reproductive organs and you should know them all well. But, we'll be focusing on the ovaries, which is where ovarian cysts form.

Uterus

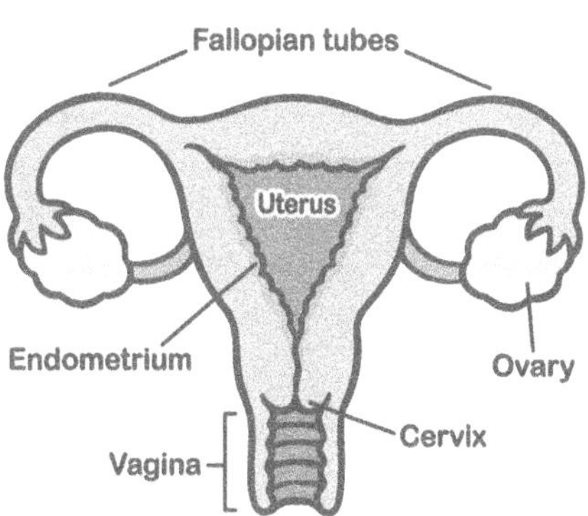

Figure 1: Gynecologic Organs

The uterus looks like a 5 to 8 centimeter (2 to 3 inch) pear. If you were to cut it in half, you'd see that it's hollow with an internal lining called the endometrium and the walls are about 1 to 2cm thick and muscular. It's located deep in the middle of the pelvis, sitting right on top of your vagina, with the bladder in front and the rectum in back. The lining or endometrium is what partly sheds every month and causes a menstrual period. This is also where a fertilized egg implants and a baby grows. More on this in a second…..

By the way, we'll be talking about sizes of different things in this book. The usual measurements you'll see on medical reports are often quoted in the "metric system". Here are the conversions you need to know. One inch is equal to 2.54 centimeters, usually abbreviated as "cm". Ten millimeters (abbreviated as "mm") is equal to one centimeter. So a millimeter is really very tiny and a centimeter is about the size of a fingernail on your hand, measured across. OK, let's move on…

Fallopian (uterine) Tubes

There are two Fallopian or uterine tubes, one is attached to each upper corner of your uterus. Fallopian tubes are hollow. If you microscopically climbed inside the open end, near the attached ovary, and kept going, you would find yourself inside the uterus. This is exactly how an egg, which comes from your ovaries during ovulation, finds its way inside the uterus to get fertilized, implant and grow into a baby.

Once it is released from one of your ovaries (at random from one side or the other), an egg takes about 4 to 5 days to travel through the Fallopian tube, helped by tiny hair-like "cilia" which push it along. Sperm will travel from the vagina, up through the cervix and uterus, and one of them will find and fertilize the egg as it is making its way through the Fallopian tube. The fertilized egg then completes its journey and lands in the uterus to implant and grow.

The reason we are even talking about this is in a book about ovarian cysts is because sometimes the fertilized egg gets stuck in the Fallopian tube. This is called an e*ctopic or tubal pregnancy* and under some conditions can mimic signs and symptoms of some ovarian cysts. The problem is that these tubal pregnancies can bleed…a LOT! So, recognizing the problem can be critical in this case or it can become life threatening.

Ovaries

There are normally two ovaries (female gonads). They are located right next to the Fallopian tubes, one on each side of your uterus. The ovaries are full of eggs (hundreds of thousands of them) in various states of maturity, from very early pre-eggs to eggs ready for fertilization. Each one is contained inside a microscopic support system called a follicle. Follicles progress from primordial ➔ primary ➔ secondary ➔ mature, before they rupture and release the egg in a process called ovulation. The ovaries also produce hormones, mainly estrogen and progesterone, but also some testosterone. Estrogen is stimulatory to some extent for mental and physical energy compared to Progesterone, which is calming on the nervous system. Testosterone, present in much lower levels than men, is essential for energy and libido or sex drive.

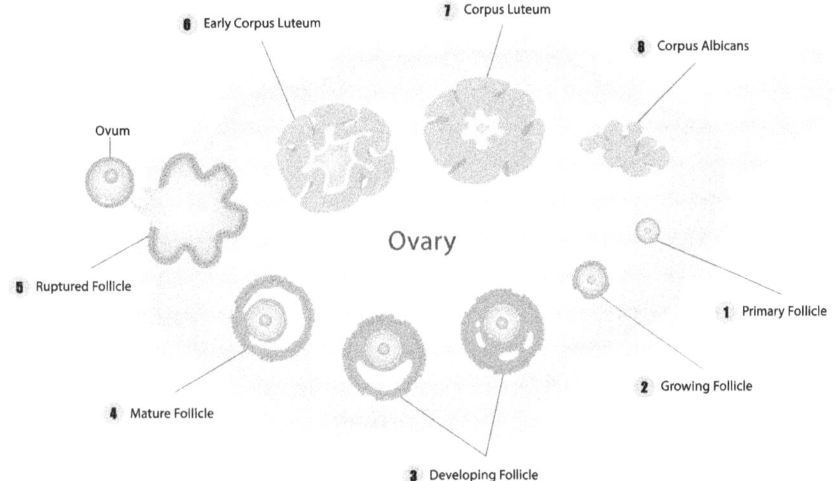

Figure 2: The ovary and follicle development stages

HORMONES

Hormones related to your normal reproductive and sexual function are called steroid hormones and the building blocks start with cholesterol. Yes, you do need healthy levels of cholesterol to keep your body functioning properly. So, cholesterol is NOT all evil. Using very complex biochemical reactions, including innumerable enzymes and co-factors, these hormones interconvert to all the hormones you need (Figure 3)…back and forth, back and forth, as needed by your body. At any point along this chain of events, something could go wrong, which affects your body in many ways including physiologic (hormone-caused) ovarian cyst formation.

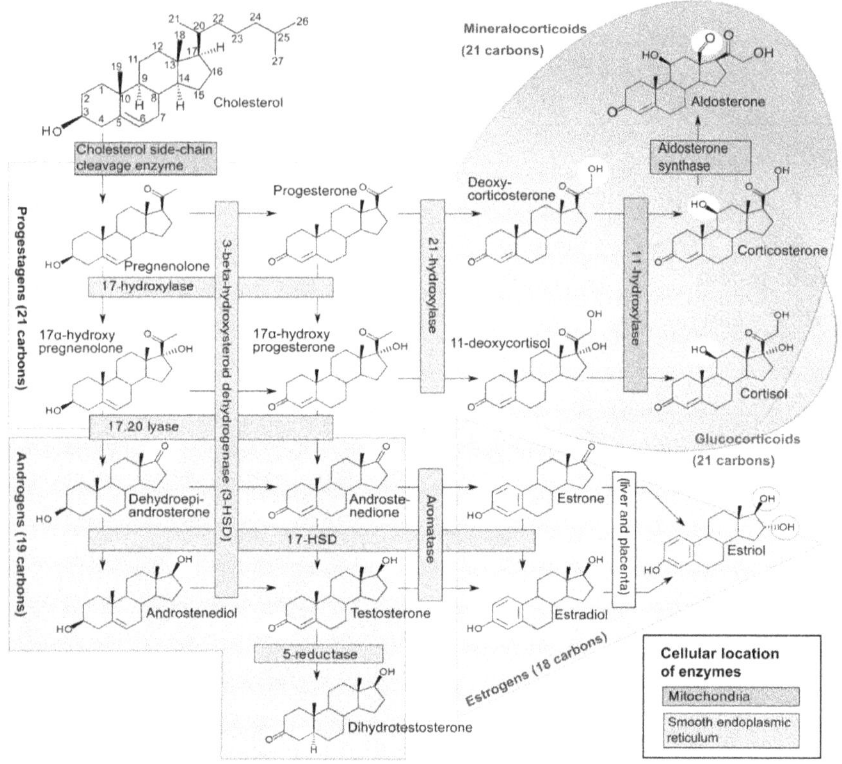

Figure 3: Sex Steroid Hormones

The chemical structure of each of these hormones looks very similar, doesn't it? The sex hormones are estrogen, progesterone and testosterone. As you can see there are a number of intermediate variations, and there are tons of others when you get into synthetic hormones which look pretty much like these, only with a few of the little "side chains" or arms off to the side of the (red) steroid rings being different. Because of this, the body sees the natural and synthetic hormones as chemically very similar, but as you shall see there are certainly some major differences.

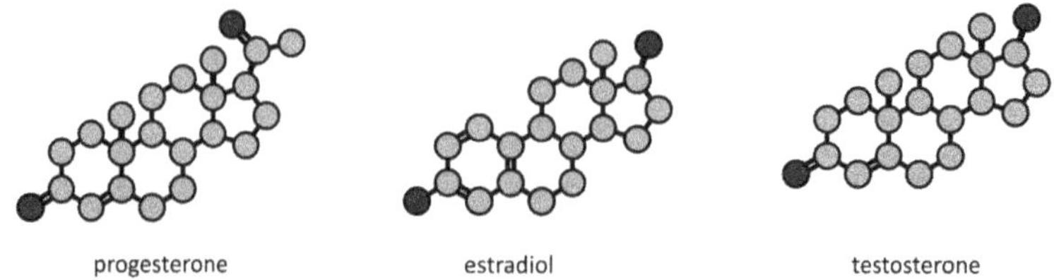

Figure 4: Estrogen, Progesterone and Testosterone

THE FEMALE REPRODUCTIVE CYCLE

As you get close to puberty, you begin to release eggs as part of a monthly period, which is called the female reproductive cycle. It's also called a monthly menstrual cycle. Once every 28 days or so, an ovary releases one egg into the Fallopian tube in a process called ovulation.

If the egg is not fertilized as it travels down the tube, it does not implant in the uterine lining (endometrium) and is instead ejected through the vagina a few days later during your menstrual flow. The bleeding during your period happens because the uterus is hormonally instructed to partly detach some of the endometrial lining. As the endometrium detaches, it tears some tiny blood vessels (capillaries) which provide blood supply to it as it thickens during the early part of the cycle. So, when this all happens you have a 4-7 day long menstrual flow, partly composed of blood and partly composed of the ejected endometrial tissue. The cycle of repeated "cleaning" and replacement of endometrial tissue repeats itself monthly if you have regular periods under normal hormonal control of the ovaries. We'll talk about that next.

The menstrual or reproductive cycle can really be divided into a closely related ovarian cycle and a uterine cycle. (Figure 5).

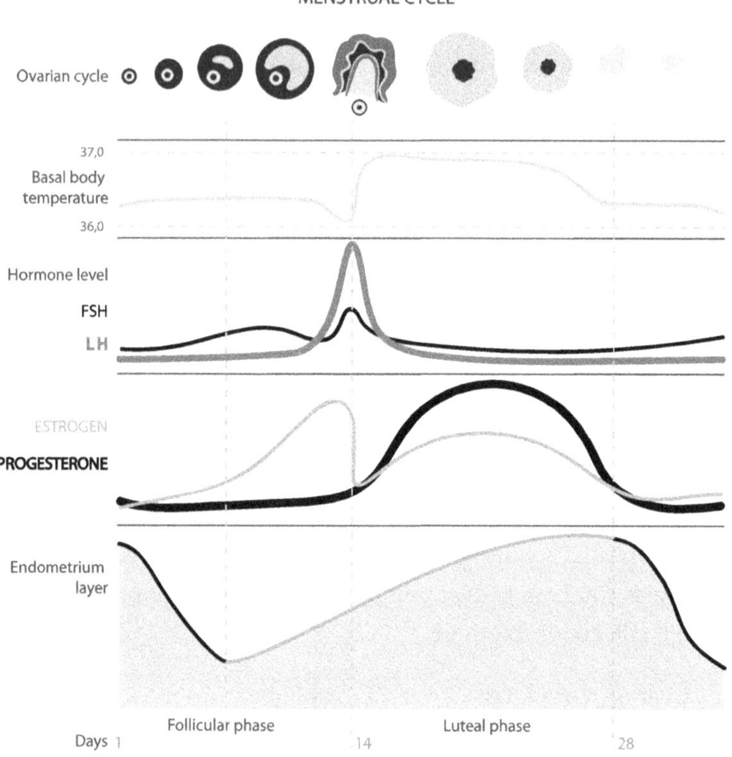

Figure 5: Ovarian and Uterine Cycles

During each uterine cycle, the endometrial lining initially builds up because of increasing levels of estrogen produced by the ovaries. During the related part of the ovarian cycle, multiple little bubbles or maturing follicles develop on the ovarian surface. Each one contains an egg, but after a week or so only one stands out as the "dominant" or mature Graffian follicle, from which the *one egg* for that cycle is released by rupture. This rupture and ovulation can cause some pain, which is called Mittelschmerz (mid-cycle pain) and can last several minutes or days. The other follicles are re-absorbed by the ovary. After the Graffian follicle releases the egg, the follicle changes how it looks and behaves. The cells in what is left of the ruptured follicle start producing progesterone and turn into what is called a Corpus Luteum. This increasing progesterone causes the uterine lining (endometrium) to get thick and well supplied with tiny blood vessels, getting ready for a fertilized egg to implant and grow.

If fertilization and implantation happen, the embryo (growing baby) and then the placenta produce a hormone called Human Chorionic Gonadotropin (hCG), which feeds back to keep the Corpus Luteum producing progesterone until the placenta takes over completely later in the pregnancy. The progesterone helps maintain the uterine lining, which keeps everything friendly inside the uterus to keep the pregnancy going.

If fertilization and implantation do NOT happen, the Corpus Luteum dies out and transforms into what is called a Corpus Albicans, which does not produce any hormones and gets absorbed by the ovary. As the progesterone levels fall, due to no more Corpus Luteum production, the endometrium responds by breaking down and forming part of the menstrual blood flow, as described above. The cycle then starts all over after the period, with the ovary starting to produce estrogen and so on, over and over on a monthly basis.

In Figure 4 you also see two other hormones listed, which are called gonadotropins. Specifically these are Follicle Simulating Hormone (FSH) and Luteinizing Hormone (LH). Without getting into too much detail beyond the scope of this book, these hormones are produced by your pituitary gland which is located at the base of your brain. They are the "regulators" which stimulate ovarian follicles to grow (FSH) and cause ovulation (LH).

All of that probably sounded very complex, but you don't need to be an expert in the anatomy, physiology and biochemistry of the reproductive cycle. If you are a health care practitioner, some of this is old-hat and over-simplified. So, it's a matter of perspective. But for the average reader, all you need to know is that it exists and you can reference the material above as you read on.

PMS OR PREMENSTRUAL SYNDROME

Many women experience hormone cycle-related physical discomfort and emotional symptoms, usually during the week prior to their menstrual period. This can continue throughout the period. Symptoms can include bloating, fatigue, backaches, sore breasts, headaches, constipation, diarrhea, acne, unusual food cravings, depression, irritability, and difficulty concentrating or handling stress. Even though it's not a focus of this book, since it's a related problem, we'll touch on some treatments for this later on.

MENOPAUSE

When your reproductive days end, menstrual cycles cease and you enter menopause, which is also known as "the change of life" or climacteric. The average age of entering menopause is around 51 to 52 years. The ovaries drastically reduce estrogen and progesterone production, which causes the reproductive system cycling to slow down and then completely stop. Estrogen circulating in your bloodstream drops by about 60% and keeps going down over the next several years. Although the ovaries stop producing estradiol (the main estrogen before menopause), you still have some estradiol and another type of estrogen (estrone) being produced by your fat cells. In this process, another type of hormone called androstenedione, which is present in many organs and tissues, gets converted into estrone, which in turn gets partly converted to estradiol. However, progesterone plummets by about 99%. The reduction in circulating hormones causes hot flashes, palpitations, anxiety, irritability, mood swings and other psychological symptoms, as well as vaginal dryness and bladder symptoms.

The mainstream medical view, based on quite a bit of research information is that the estrogen fall-off is what causes the symptoms of menopause. But the truth is menopause is still relatively poorly understood in terms of why symptoms occur. For example, the alternative viewpoint is that it is the progesterone reduction that causes most of the havoc in your body at menopause. This has not been proven, but is often quoted in books you may read as "estrogen dominance." During the final five or so years prior to menopause, due to irregular hormone production by the ovaries, cycles start getting irregular as they become less frequent.

Menopause can occur "early" (between ages 40 and 50) and is defined as "premature" if it occurs before the age of 40. This is very unusual, but may be caused by other diseases like autoimmune disorders, thyroid disease, and diabetes.

Normally, menopause comes about naturally with gradual reduction in hormones over the years. However, if your uterus and ovaries are removed before menopause you will also feel the changes and symptoms. These symptoms can be more drastic because you feel the immediate or abrupt drop in hormone levels when the ovaries are removed.

Other than symptoms, how do you know if you are going into menopause? Menopause can be diagnosed by measuring the levels of follicle stimulating hormone (FSH) and luteinizing hormone (LH), which both increase and stay elevated right around and after menopause.

OK, now that you have the basics down, let's start with the most common ovarian cysts. These develop in most women at some point in their life, are the most treatable by natural means and are generally called "physiologic" or "functional" cysts. They are so named because they usually come and go under normal physiologic hormonal influence during your reproductive years. These cysts do not occur after menopause, although a physiologic cyst formed right around menopause may essentially fail to pop or resolve and stay with you potentially for the rest of your life. Usually these do not cause problems, but there are issues that can occur. Read on.

Physiologic or Functional Cysts

FOLLICULAR CYSTS

Follicular cysts are hands down the most frequent types of cysts that occur in the ovaries. These cysts can often occur more than one per ovary and measure from a few millimeters (tiny) to a 15 centimeter (6 inch) cyst, or even larger. Any normal ovarian follicle during any menstrual cycle may turn into a physiologic cyst. Cysts are usually about an inch, or between 2.5 and 3 centimeters in size (remember those measurement size conversions we talked about in the introduction).

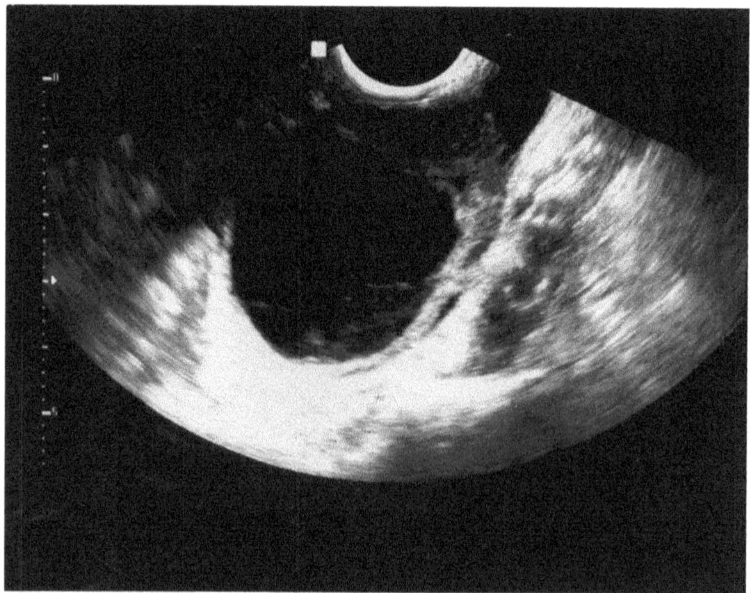

Figure 5b: 3cm (a little less than an inch) Simple Cyst on Ultrasound

Follicular cysts are not "tumors", which are actual abnormal cell growths or lumps on the ovary. Follicular cysts are simply thin fluid-filled little sacs, called cysts, which develop from follicles (tiny sacs which hold eggs) and are under the influence of hormone fluctuation (gonadotropins: FSH and LH) in your body. As we shall see, some of these fluctuations are normal, but some are not. Most cysts grow because of a temporary change or alteration in normal physiology of the ovaries. Normally, after ovulation or if the ovulation does not occur, the follicle or sac simply gets reabsorbed by the ovary. But this follicle sac can also swell up with fluid, forming a cyst. These cysts might last just a short time (hours or days) and pop or they can keep swelling or stay the same size and simply refuse to go away. It's truly all over the map and we'll be covering all of these possibilities.

It's important to keep hammering on the following point. Before deciding upon what treatment is needed, it is crucial to understand the difference between different types of cysts and to understand that some of them are not cysts at all. Some are actually tumors that are hollow, so they look like cysts on an ultrasound or other scans. What you read here will help you understand what your doctor needs to do to make sure you do not have ovarian tumors, benign or malignant (cancerous). Once that distinction is made, it is much easier, and safer, to find a natural approach to treating the different types of the more common physiologic cysts.

Most often, follicular cysts are found in younger women in their reproductive years. They are rarely found in children prior to onset of menses and also should not occur after menopause under most circumstances. Again, the reason is that these are physiologic cysts which come and go under the influence of fluctuating hormones; something which does not normally occur before the onset of menses or after menopause. However, sometimes a cyst may go undetected in the peri-menopausal years and stays with you into the menopausal years. Some of these never go away, but do not grow and are not dangerous. In fact one large study found that about 15% of postmenopausal women have simple cysts (physiologic cysts that never went away) ranging from about half a centimeter to about 5 cm. Physiologic functional cysts can also occur in pregnancy and right after pregnancy, but they are of a special type that we'll cover later.

A blood test, called CA125, is often obtained when there is some concern that an ovarian cystic mass might be malignant or cancerous. It is a very inaccurate test, but a value less than 35 U/ml is considered normal in most laboratories. In the reproductive years it is generally not very useful because almost anything, any inflammation, including a bad migraine headache or even a period, can cause CA125 to be elevated or abnormal. However, it is often obtained anyway because if it is very high (100's or 1000's) that may signal trouble. Pregnancy itself can cause it to be elevated, so during a pregnancy it is not very helpful. However, CA125 tends to normalize after the fourth month of pregnancy. If it is extremely high during pregnancy, like the high 100s or 1000s, then there might be reason to be concerned. Mainly, when it is elevated in the postmenopausal years, in the presence of an ovarian mass, it is more often a sign of trouble. This means possible cancer, but not in all cases. Again, keep in mind, any inflammation (e.g. arthritis of intestinal upset) can cause it to rise.

By the way, women who have a rare condition called cystic fibrosis tend to develop more follicular cysts. If you have this condition, you would know it by the time you reached puberty, usually by having major lung infection troubles.

How do you know if you have a follicular cyst? The best test is a pelvic ultrasound. Follicular cysts look like simple little thin-walled fluid filled balloons or sacs. They are usually located on the surface of the ovary, so multiple little cysts may be seen and look like tiny domes on the surface of the solid part of the ovary.

Why do follicular cysts form? The short answer is although we can explain what is going on (read above regarding hormone influence), we don't really know why it happens only some of the time or why it may happen on a regular basis in only some women. Follicular cysts usually form when a follicle that is about to release an egg, by rupturing, does not rupture. So, the egg remains stuck in its protective little fluid sac. Sometimes the follicle is not mature and does not even contain a mature egg, but the protective little follicle sac grows and also does not get reabsorbed or rupture. Finally, sometimes ovulation DOES occur but the follicle sac re-seals quickly and swells up with fluid just like a follicle that never ruptured. The end result of any of these possibilities is the same kind of follicular cyst, which will likely go away over time.

Why might you have abnormal periods when you have follicular ovarian cysts? Well, these cysts are lined with "granulosa cells" that produce estrogen during egg development and maturation. Sometimes, these estrogen producing "granulosa cells" keep producing estrogen and this can cause abnormal uterine bleeding. Why? Because the uterus is "confused." Its normal hormonal cycling is interrupted and the internal lining of the uterus (endometrium), which normally sheds or comes out with blood during a regular period, can start to partly shed in between periods. Most often there is a "missed period" in someone who has had regular periods before, followed by several heavy bleeding episodes over the coming weeks. After that, assuming new cysts don't grow, the periods go back to normal.

A follicular cyst can enlarge over time because fluid continues to accumulate inside or it can bleed inside the cyst, causing it to expand. The cyst is not really "growing", but it can appear like it is getting bigger when a repeat ultrasound is done. Growth is often used by surgeons to determine if a cyst might really be a tumor and, in particular, one that is cancerous. So, this is an important point to discuss with your doctor when considering surgery for "an enlarging ovarian cyst or mass." The devil is in the details and requires expert review.

How are follicular cysts found? Most women have small cysts coming and going every month, or every other month, which do not normally cause symptoms. So, when a routine pelvic examination is done or an ultrasound ordered for some other reason, a cyst on the ovary can be a surprise finding. Keep on mind that this is not unusual.

Because they are very thin and fragile, follicular cysts may easily leak or break on their own or during sex or vigorous exercise or a pelvic examination. Leaking follicular cysts may cause temporary pelvic pain or tenderness or may not cause any symptoms at all. It is not known why some women are more irritated inside by leaking cyst fluid than others. When these cysts rupture, they can also bleed, which can also cause irritation and pain. However, unless you have a blood clotting disorder, are on anticoagulant medications (e.g. Warfarin, Coumadin, Heparin) or aspirin/ibuprofen or herbals/supplements (e.g. Vitamin E, Ginko Biloba) that can thin out your blood, the bleeding is rarely severe. On the other hand, a large ruptured follicular cyst can certainly lead to an emergency surgery due to severe pain and/or heavy internal bleeding. Again, this is rare.

What are the most common symptoms of follicular cysts? In addition to the pain from fluid or blood leaking out and the abnormal uterine bleeding (abnormal periods), other symptoms can occur. These complications can occur with any ovarian cyst or tumor as it grows. Any ovarian mass can cause a vague pressure sensation, constipation due to pressure on the rectum, urinary frequency or urgency due to pressure on the bladder and severe pain due to twisting of the ovary and cyst around itself (called torsion). This last symptom is a surgical emergency and happens because the cyst is just large enough to flip on itself (usually greater than 5cm in size), causing the ovarian blood vessels and ligaments that hold the ovary in place to twist like a pretzel. This type of pain is usually severe, very colicky in that it comes and goes repeatedly, and causes nausea and vomiting. It's the kind of pain that causes you to double over, and even curl up into a fetal position. But then it suddenly can release, until it happens again minutes or hours later. This can cycle over and over. If that is happening to you, it is prudent to head over to the closest emergency room.

How are follicular cysts treated? Because these cysts come and go very often, most will go away on their own just by waiting. In other words, if there are no symptoms or they are fairly minor, you can just wait it out and repeat an ultrasound after a menstrual cycle or two. Most of these cysts simply get reabsorbed or silently leak, causing no symptoms.

What happens if the cyst does not go away? While your doctor can take a good professional educated guess, there is no way to know for sure if the persistent ovarian cyst is a physiologic cyst or an ovarian tumor. The problem is that the pelvic examination findings or how fast the cyst enlarged (if it did) do not always help. Ultrasound of the pelvis, especially using a special vaginal probe, can help measure the cyst and take a close look at what it is made up of. Ovarian masses can be simple cysts (nothing inside the fluid sac) or complex, meaning there are both cystic fluid areas and solid parts. Complex cysts (solid parts within) are rarely physiologic and most will end up requiring surgery to remove them. Most but not all of these are "tumors" which simply means a "growth." These are usually benign (not malignant) but a small percentage can be cancer. If you have a family history of breast or ovarian cancer, your risk of having a malignant tumor may be higher and this is something important to discuss with your doctor.

When the cyst remains the same size for more than 8 to 10 weeks, or gets bigger, a tumor (benign or cancerous) of the ovary is possible. The only other scan that might help in this case is an "MRI", which can help determine if you might have an endometrioma. This is a special type of benign cyst which occurs when you have a condition called endometriosis, and we will discuss this a little later in this book.

What about birth control pills? Do they help treat functional follicular cysts? The short answer is no, they only help prevent future cysts from forming. How does this work? Oral contraceptive pills decrease the amount of hormones that stimulate the ovary (gonadotropins: FSH and LH) coming from your pituitary gland. By reducing the gonadotropin levels, complete egg follicle development and ovulation does not occur and you don't get pregnant. Basically, what this all means is that your body is "tricked" into thinking it is already pregnant, so your ovaries think it is unnecessary to ovulate. Oral contraceptives are not 100% effective in preventing pregnancy, but they are in a pretty high 99% range. This is EXACTLY how they prevent functional ovarian cysts from forming too. No ovulation and no follicle, means no cyst. So, your doctor may still give you "the pill" to prevent future cysts from forming. To say that birth control pills do not work to prevent cysts is like saying they don't prevent pregnancy. Obviously, they do, and there is good scientific proof for it. However, there might be other issues and there are potential side effects to any medication. More on this later.

CORPUS LUTEUM CYSTS

Another type of physiologic or functional cyst is known as a Corpus Luteum Cyst, or CLC for short. These are less frequent than a follicular cyst, but can cause more problems and emergencies. There are technically two types of cysts in this category: mature functioning corpus luteum and a CLC, although for practical purposes they are treated the same and can cause the same problems. I'm just giving you the full scoop so that you can talk about all of this with your doc using some of the same language they might use.

As part of your normal ovarian cycle, the Corpus Luteum initially grows and then stops or slows down its main function of producing hormones, then gets absorbed as the next cycle starts. Normally a Corpus Luteum lasts, very predictably, only 14 days. If it gets to 3 cm in size or larger, it is termed a Corpus Luteum Cyst (CLC). The reason I am even mentioning all of this is that a 2cm cystic-looking corpus luteum may not technically be called a CLC by your doctor, but if it does not go away normally it continues to produce hormones (mainly a lot of progesterone) for a prolonged time of weeks to months. This can lead to menstrual irregularities like spotting because the uterus is "confused" by too much progesterone and starts to shed its lining irregularly, often after a missed period or two. If the Corpus Luteum then eventually stops producing the progesterone, a heavy period may also result. This may seem like you are pregnant initially, because of the missed period, but the pregnancy test would be negative.

Normally the Corpus Luteum develops from a mature egg follicle (called a Graffian Follicle) after the egg is released (ovulation). Within a few days of ovulation, tiny blood vessels (capillaries) grow into the wall of the Corpus Luteum. These tiny capillaries can break and bleed a small amount into the central part of the Corpus Luteum, creating a blood-filled small cyst. Normally the blood is absorbed over the next few days and the Corpus Luteum is normally absorbed by the ovary, in a process called involution. If bleeding into the Corpus Luteum is excessive, then the central cyst part gets bigger and if the pressure builds rapidly the cyst can rupture, causing bleeding and pelvic pain. If it does not rupture, it is now called a CLC. These can actually grow up to 15cm in size, which is pretty large, approximating the size of a cantaloupe or small melon. Also, as the blood inside the cyst gets absorbed, a thin fluid accumulates inside the cyst to replace it. The CLC often becomes hormonally inactive and is then technically called a Corpus Albicans Cyst, which usually gets absorbed slowly.

Why is all this detail important? Because, as I keep emphasizing, a cyst is not a cyst is not a cyst. They are *all different*, with different biological behavior that determines the kind of problems you will experience and what kind of treatment will work and what won't. You should also learn and know some of the terms that your doctor is throwing around or terms you should ask about. So, for example, a persistent Corpus Lutuem and early CLC may cause hormonally related irregular periods, but a Corpus Albicans cyst will not. On the other hand, a Corpus Albicans, like many other cysts, can twist on itself (called torsion) and cause severe crampy, colicky pelvic pain.

As mentioned above, if a pregnancy occurs after ovulation and fertilization, a Corpus Luteum of pregnancy normally stays about 2 to 3cm in size and is hormonally active, supporting the uterine lining (endometrium) and making the uterus a friendly place for your baby to grow.

The CLC may be small, usually in the 3-5 cm size range, but they can cause serious problems, often from internal bleeding and pain due to rupture. Sometimes the bleeding and pain are severe enough that emergency surgery is recommended.

So, how do you know if you have a CLC? A missed period followed by some spotting, one sided pelvic pain and a pelvic examination which finds a tender ovarian mass suggest that a persistent Corpus Luteum or CLC is the culprit. However, it is important to make sure a pregnancy test is ordered because these same findings may be there because of an ectopic pregnancy (tubal pregnancy). An ultrasound may not be able to tell these two apart and the treatment would be completely different. Although beyond the scope of this book, let me just say that ectopic pregnancies are treated very differently, often with surgery or a strong medicine (chemotherapy) called Methotrexate. So, if the pregnancy test is negative, these findings are most likely related to a Corpus Luteum/CLC and not an ectopic pregnancy. One other possibility is an endometrioma type of cyst and we'll touch on that later.

When a Corpus Luteum or CLC ruptures, the amount of bleeding and/or pain may cause this to be a surgical emergency. Also, sometimes the internal bleeding is severe enough to require a blood transfusion. These fragile cysts can rupture easily, often just because of a pelvic exam or sex. So, if you take aspirin, herbal/supplements or blood thinners (like Coumadin or Heparin), or have any medical condition which causes you to bruise easily (blood clotting disorder) the chances of heavy bleeding internally may be increased. This type of bleeding is most likely to happen during your 3rd or 4th week of the menstrual cycle.

Unfortunately, one third of women (33%) who have a problem with bleeding from a Corpus Luteum or a CLC will have it happen again, possibly over and over. Just like they work to prevent follicular cysts, oral contraceptives are effective in preventing ovulation and thus preventing the Corpus Luteum from ever forming.

CLC Symptoms

Sudden severe lower abdominal pain, which does not go away, is the main symptom of a CLC rupture. After hours or days it may let up, but the blood and fluid from the rupture can irritate your insides and cause a lesser amount of pain for up to a week. This is much different from the pressure and gnawing feeling of a cyst that is pressing on other organs in the pelvis. Also, it is different from the pain of torsion (cyst and ovary twisting on itself) which is also severe, but colicky and crampy, causing nausea. To repeat, torsion will literally grab you and double you over, but then relaxes for minutes to an hour, only to do it again. I'm repeating this to make sure you know that if this is going on, the emergency room is a good idea.

By the way, pelvic pain with or without ovarian cysts being present does not mean the pain is coming from a gynecologic organ. In other words, there are other things down there in your pelvis. Pain can be caused by bladder problems, large or small bowel problems and, importantly, possibly an appendicitis. The symptoms of appendicitis may come on just like a combination of a ruptured cyst or torsion and may be dull initially or sharp, causing you to double over and be very nauseated. Keep this in mind because appendicitis is also usually a surgical emergency, so it is best handled before a big abscess and infection occur.

If a CLC keep rupturing over an over again with repeat cycles, the blood irritates and can scar your internal skin-like lining called the peritoneum. With repeated irritation, scars form and are called adhesions, because they cause adherence or stickiness between organs in the pelvis, like the bladder, rectum, uterus, ovaries and colon. When the intestines move, like they constantly normally do, they tug on the adhesions and cause pain. This is a chronic dull aching or crampy pain usually and can't easily be remedied because adhesions tend to stay. If you have surgery to cut adhesions, the scars or adhesions tend to re-form. Although there is no guarantee, there are some things the surgeon can do that might minimize this like putting a film-like protective substances on to the area of surgery and performing the surgery using minimally invasive techniques.

The most life-threatening complication of a Corpus Luteum or CLC rupture is internal bleeding. Sometimes ultrasound or other scans can help find out if you are bleeding, but as an alternative a doctor may put a needle in through the vagina into a space between the uterus and rectum. This is the lowest part of your pelvis so if there is any bleeding or fluid accumulating inside you, it would pool there. The procedure is called a culdocentesis and can help find out if it is fluid or blood that is the problem, but can be very painful.

If surgery is necessary because of bleeding, it is often possible to do it through a minimally invasive laparoscope (band-aid surgery). Usually the ovary does not have to be removed. Only the cyst is removed and the bleeding is stopped.

If the cyst is NOT ruptured, there is no bleeding or torsion, then it is reasonable to avoid surgery and "wait it out." Why? Because surgery, no matter how small, can cause scars or adhesions (internal scars) to form. You want to avoid surgery if your doctor thinks it is safe based on all of the things you just read about.

THECA LUTEIN CYSTS

The least common type of physiologic or functional cysts are called Theca Lutein Cysts or TLC. The key difference is that these are usually multiple, on both ovaries, and occur all at the same time. Each of these cysts can be 1cm to 10cm in size, so if there are multiple cysts the ovaries can be massively enlarged; up to 20-30cm on both sides. How does this happen? The answer is over-stimulation of the ovaries or increased sensitivity of the ovaries to those hormones your pituitary gland produces called gonadotropins, LH and FSH. We covered these in the first chapter. Gonadotropins are also sometimes given artificially to women who are trying to get pregnant but need some help to produce ovulation. When these cysts occur, there is either too much gonadotropin hormone circulating or the ovaries are too sensitive to the hormone.

Cells in the normal human placenta produce human chorionic gonadotropin (hCG). This is the hormone that is tested for in a pregnancy test. Because of this additional gonadotropin, TLC may be found during pregnancy, most often when there is a large placenta due to twins, diabetes or Rh blood sensitization. Also, rare conditions like a molar pregnancy (an abnormal pregnancy where only the placenta, not the baby forms) and a related malignancy called choriocarcinoma, can produce hCG in high levels and cause TLC to form. Occasionally TLC can be found in normal pregnancies, probably because the ovaries are too sensitive to the hCG hormone.

In most cases, Theca Lutein Cysts do not get huge. But if they do, they can certainly cause a pressure sensation in the pelvic area. There may also be some "free fluid" seen on ultrasound in your pelvis because some of the cysts can be leaking or rupturing. This free fluid is called "ascites" and, with the massively enlarged ovaries, may look like cancer on scans. It is not, but can cause quite a scare. Either the fluid can be removed by a needle and checked for malignant (cancer) cells or a second opinion regarding how the scan looks can help make sure that it is not cancer. Rarely an ovary with a large TLC cluster can also twist on itself (torsion), causing severe pain. It can also leak, rupture or bleed. In most cases after pregnancy is over, or artificial ovarian stimulation with gonadotropin is stopped, the cysts slowly go away by themselves over several months. If these cysts don't completely go away, it may mean that you have a tumor which may need to be removed surgically.

SUMMARY: Follicular cysts, Corpus Luteum cysts and Theca Lutein cysts are all "physiologic" or "functional" because they are under hormonal control. They are very common and usually do not cause problems. However, they can leak twist or rupture and cause severe pain, sometimes even requiring emergency surgery. These cysts are unpredictable but can often be prevented using medical and natural means, as you will discover later in this book.

Endometrioma or Endometriotic Cyst

If you have *endometriosis*, the chances are very high that it will be growing on your ovaries, forming cystic masses called endometriomas. Endometriosis is a benign (not cancer) condition or disease where cells and tissue of a similar type that are normally found inside the uterus (endometrium) start growing outside the uterus and mostly inside your pelvis. The pelvis is the area that your ovaries and bladder and rectum are located. The good news is that even though 70% of women with endometriosis have it growing on their ovaries, only 5% actually develop a significant size endometriotic cyst that actually causes problems like pain or infertility.

An endometrioma forms when a cystic area on the ovary, lined by glands that are like the ones inside your uterine lining, starts bleeding into itself on a regular monthly "period" schedule. The blood has nowhere to go, so it accumulates in the cyst and the endometrioma slowly gets larger and larger with each period. The blood inside gets old and turns into a thick brown pasty fluid, which is why these are also called "chocolate cysts." Endometriomas can be tiny or can enlarge to be 20cm in size or larger, and are often found on both ovaries.

Until they become larger and leak or rupture, endometriomas might cause no symptoms at all. However, due to leaks of this old blood from an endometrioma or since the endometriosis grows in multiple areas, pelvic pain, painful sex, bowel symptoms (including bloating), and infertility often occur. When endometriomas leak or rupture, the old blood containing "chocolate fluid" causes severe inflammation and scarring. The scars that form, called adhesions, cause a lot of organs to stick together densely. This includes the ovaries, uterus, Fallopian tubes, bladder, rectum and small intestine. In really severe cases, when surgery is required, it can be extremely difficult for the surgeon to determine what is what, increasing the risk of injury to one or more of these areas and organs. For best results, an über-expert surgeon is required for endometriosis surgery, and we'll cover more of that later.

How do you know if you have endometriosis and/or endometriomas? The only way to know for sure is surgery and biopsies. There are no accurate blood tests to make the diagnosis yet, but this may be coming soon based on ongoing research. However, ultrasound can be of help in some cases. When in doubt, an MRI scan can be used to quite accurately confirm that the mass is or is not an endometrioma.

How are endometriomas treated? In most cases, the bigger question is how is endometriosis treated? This is because the symptoms of bloating, pain or presence of infertility are due to the disease, not just the endometrioma. This book's focus is on cysts, so I'm not going to dwell on endometriosis information too much, which can fill up several books by itself. In general, endometriosis is treated by a combination of hormonal options and surgical excision. The outcomes are best when the diagnosis is made early, which can be in the teen years, and treated appropriately. Surgical excision is usually best left to experienced specialty trained gynecologists (endo excision surgeons) and/or gynecologic oncologists, who do very advanced surgery including cancer excision. Endometriosis can mimic ovarian cancer in terms of difficulty of removal and, rarely (~1.5%), endometriosis can become cancerous itself. Even though 1.5% seems like a tiny number, since there are over 9 million women afflicted with endometriosis, this means tens of thousands may have cancer too. So, the more über-expert surgeon you can find, the more you will like your results. Most often the worst cases are best handled by gynecologic oncologists who are faced with very similar surgical challenges found in ovarian cancer. In both diseases the anatomy is often severely distorted, requiring advanced knowledge of anatomy. Removal of as much disease as possible is the common goal between endometriosis excision and ovarian debulking surgery. Endo tends to recur, so the best surgery up front leads to better results in the long run.

As far as what to do about an endometrioma, smaller ones that are causing no symptoms generally will do you no harm. As long as you are not concerned about getting pregnant (infertility), you can certainly wait. The problem is that endometriomas will continue to bleed and get bigger with each period you have.

How fast is hard to say, but when an endometrioma leaks or ruptures it will cause pain and scarring which can be VERY difficult to treat. Unfortunately, it is the thin walled small endometrioma which tends to leak or rupture. So, it is hard to recommend waiting with no treatment at all. Most often, medical treatment using several hormonal approaches is used, followed by surgery. But sometimes it is mainly surgery. The surgery and what is removed depends upon a complex decision-making process which includes whether or not you want to keep possible pregnancy as a future option and how damaged your reproductive organs are. This requires a highly individualized patient-surgeon discussion.

The primary treatment strategies for endometriosis and endometriomas are similar worldwide, stretching out as far as China. While prevention may be possible to some extent with diet, weight management, and some herbals, this is not a disease that can be effectively treated with herbals or medications alone. More on this later in the treatment options chapters.

PolyCystic Ovary Syndrome (PCOS)

The term "PCOS" or Polycystic Ovarian Syndrome is perhaps one of the most abused terms involving ovarian cysts. It does NOT simply mean that you have multiple cysts on your ovaries. In fact, you may or may not have any significant size cysts on your ovaries and no ovarian symptoms at all with this syndrome. Basically, PCOS is a very complex physiologic disorder which involves multiple body systems and processes. These processes lead to irregular ovulation and, in about 60-70% of women, cyst formation. But looking at the cysts as the primary problem in PCOS is kind of like looking at the wrong end of a horse. You could get kicked and hurt badly by ignoring the main problems.

Although having cysts on the ovary does NOT mean you have PCOS, the bad news is that PCOS affects up to 10% of all reproductive age women. So, while cystic ovaries may have caused you to look into what is going on with you, it is very important to make sure that you don't have PCOS. If you are diagnosed with PCOS, ovarian cysts are possibly the least of your worries. On the other hand, physiologic or functional cyst formation, without the other findings of PCOS, may depend at least partly on similar biochemical processes gone astray. In other words, there may be some overlap in how these cysts form and some PCOS related remedies may work for you, even if you don't have a diagnosis of PCOS. This last statement is certainly not exact or proven, but something to think about as we get into remedies, cures and prevention strategies later in the book.

Irregular ovulation in PCOS may have started way back when your periods started (menarche) or they may have begun later, usually by the early twenties. By then it should be apparent if you have true PCOS or not, based on biochemical blood tests.

The second most common finding in PCOS is too high of a "male" hormone level in your system. These "male" hormones are called androgens. A small amount of these hormones is normally produced by your ovaries and adrenal glands. This is just as normal as some "female" hormones, in small amounts, in men. But in PCOS the androgen hormone levels are much higher than normal for a woman. The most common type of male hormone or androgen that is elevated in PCOS is Testosterone, a particularly strong androgen. At the same time that Testosterone is elevated, Progesterone, which is necessary for normal cycling and egg release is low.

Some signs of elevated Testosterone include facial and body hair overgrowth, oily skin, weight gain, some irregular skin color changes, and persistent acne which does not respond well to usual medications. You might also detect deepening of the voice and/or enlargement of the clitoris. As testosterone levels climb, so does the libido or sex drive.

Women who have PCOS often have other health related issues including obesity (over 50% of PCOS patients are overweight), insulin resistance/diabetes, abnormal lipid levels in the blood stream, cardiovascular disease and endometrial (uterine) cancer. It used to be thought that these were just coincidental, but they are actually highly related issues.

I don't want to simplify this complex disorder too much. Mainly you should understand that PCOS exists and that it is more complex than just formation of physiologic cysts. But, for example, in PCOS both the ovaries and adrenal glands (near your kidneys) produce androgens (testosterone and related hormones). When you gain weight your body becomes somewhat resistant to insulin and you start entering a pre-diabetic state, or possibly even start developing diabetes (diabetes mellitus). High insulin levels actually stimulate more ovarian and adrenal androgen production and reduce the blood levels of "sex hormone binding globulin" (SHBG). This globulin normally holds on to hormones like testosterone (an androgen). When SHBG is reduced, more Testosterone is "free" and available to cause male-like findings like facial hair overgrowth, oily skin, deepened voice, found in PCOS.

While all that already sounds totally complicated, it's actually not that "simple". Your fat cells, of which you have 25-30 billion or more, contain an enzyme called an aromatase. This enzyme can convert the androgens produced by the ovaries and adrenal into estrone…another type of estrogen which naturally occurs in your body. The fatter you are, the more estrone you produce. And guess what? The estrone type of estrogen actually ADDS to the insulin resistance problem. What happens then? You get even fatter! It's a vicious cycle and this is why the PCOS story is extremely complex and requires a LOT of attention to detail to treat properly. More on this in a minute. I should also mention that PCOS may run in families, so look around at close relatives and what problems they may be having.

Since PCOS is a complicated problem, treatment for PCOS is also very complex and is well beyond the scope of this book. However, in a nutshell, the cornerstone of treatment is controlled weight loss with a good nutrition and exercise program (reduces insulin resistance and estrone production by fat cells), prescription medications or laser surgery for the excessive hair growth (often Cyproterone, alone or in combination with ethinyl estradiol, and spironolactone) and active monitoring and treatment of impaired glucose tolerance and diabetes. A common prescription medication used in PCOS treatment is Metformin, which is a drug which helps overcome insulin resistance. In addition, if fertility concerns were what brought you to the doctor, there are additional medications required to help you ovulate and conceive. The cornerstone of all this, which you can certainly start yourself, is a *healthy lifestyle transformation*. The rest is very complex and requires detailed medical management.

While there are some natural options for treatment of PCOS you can explore with a naturopathic or homeopathic doctor, the nature and scope of potentially severe health problems is so complex you would do yourself a favor to work with a mainstream allopathic or osteopathic physician who knows how to manage PCOS specifically. Usually this is either an allopathic or osteopathic endocrinologist or an obstetrician-gynecologist who specializes in infertility.

Again, the focus of this book is not on PCOS, but here are a few tips. First, if you are inclined to explore the natural path, please at least get fully evaluated so that you stay out of serious health trouble. Second, based on published research from China and Japan, two of the more promising natural herbal support remedies are "unkei-to" (also known as "wen-jing-tang") and "tiangui fang" (Hou). Third, acupuncture has been used with some effectiveness for cyst resolution as well as symptom control, which is mainly pain.

"Ovarian Cyst" Treatment Strategies

As you hopefully are now realizing, the best treatment plan depends on what exactly the ovarian cyst type is or what it is most likely to be. It is super critical to keep in mind, a cyst is not a cyst is not a cyst. Which type it is can be crucial to your successful treatment, and to prevention. So, determining what this cyst is most likely to be is JOB #1. The problem is that it is not always possible to tell for sure from an examination and ultrasound. This is where it is crucial to have a good doctor to review the possibilities with you depending on your specific situation and to develop the best strategy for you!

Strategies range from "presumed" physiologic cyst treatment, which depends on ultrasound and sometimes on blood tests, to definite surgery for tumors or cancers of the ovary. Part one of a safe plan is to determine whether or not you actually have a physiologic cyst. Fortunately, compared to physiologic cysts, a cancer or even a benign tumor that looks like a simple cyst is far less common. Also, we are talking about the management of the cysts themselves here. Other health problems, like the ones in PCOS, discussed above, are in addition to these points we're about to go through here.

So, here are some general strategies that your doctor may suggest:

(1) If you are in your reproductive years and a simple cyst (i.e. nothing apparently inside of it other than fluid on scan) is found on ultrasound or examination and there are no symptoms, it is usually reasonable to repeat the ultrasound in 6 to 10 weeks to look for changes. Most of the time, if it is a physiologic cyst, it will go away on its own. If it doesn't, it may mean you have a "tumor" and you may be headed for surgery, especially if it keeps growing or if more solid parts are seen growing inside of the cystic area.

(2) If the cyst is complex (has solid parts) or is more than 10cm in size, surgery is the usual recommendation, because it is probably a tumor and not a physiologic cyst. Tumors will not go away on their own like physiologic cysts, which quite often will. In most cases a tumor is benign (not cancer), but it will continue to grow. So, there is usually no percentage is waiting to the point where it may be harder to safely remove. Also, if a close relative has or has had ovarian, colon or breast cancer it is especially urgent to discuss the findings with your doctor and determine the plan, which usually will include surgery. This family history may mean your risk of cancer is higher.

(3) The CA-125 blood test, which is mainly used to monitor how well treatment is going in patients with known ovarian cancer, may be ordered. In the reproductive years it is rarely helpful because, as mentioned before, it can be abnormal due to a lot of non-cancer inflammatory conditions, even a bad period or migraine. However, in the postmenopausal years it can help make the decision as to whether or not surgery is needed. After menopause an elevated CA-125 in the presence of an enlarged ovary, even a simple looking cyst, is more likely to be related to an ovarian cancer. Don't panic if it is, because it may still be a benign tumor or endometriosis. However, surgery should be the next step in most cases.

Another newer blood test called the OVA-1 is a combination test of multiple markers like CA-125, and is reported as a risk range for both premenopausal and postmenopausal women with an ovarian cystic mass. Depending on the range it is helpful to determine if a cancer specialist, a gynecologic oncologist, should be involved or not. This test is FDA approved to determine who the surgeon should be, not whether or not to perform surgery. This is because it is not 100% accurate either, so one would not want to be falsely reassured based on an inaccurately low risk result.

(4) An ultrasound is key to the evaluation. If a cyst is not a "simple" or clear balloon-like sac on the ultrasound picture, this may be a warning sign. Complexities in a cystic ovarian mass, including solid areas or thick dividing membranes called septations, strongly suggest that it is NOT a physiologic cyst. An additional feature of ultrasound is the ability to measure blood flow in the area of an ovarian cyst. This is called Color Flow Doppler which can see excessive abnormal blood flow, common in tumors (not cysts). However, while it is widely used and sometimes helps, it is not really very accurate in determining whether or not a cystic ovarian mass might be a cancerous tumor.

If an ovarian cyst is found during pregnancy, and it is simple on ultrasound, especially with a normal CA125, repeat ultrasound in four to six weeks is a very reasonable plan. Often these are Theca Lutein (TL) cysts, are related to pregnancy, and will go away on their own after delivery. However, repeat ultrasound is a must in order to make sure that the cyst or cysts have gone away.

(5) If a cyst is found around the time of, or after, menopause, it should be surgically removed if it is large (greater than 10cm), complex or if the CA125 blood test is abnormal. Again, anything under a CA125 level of 35 is considered normal. If an OVA-1 is elevated, then a gynecologic oncologist should be involved in the surgery. If it is a smaller simple cyst (5 cm or so) and the CA125 test is normal, it is OK to wait and repeat the ultrasound in about 6 weeks. A cyst will not go away after menopause, because all of the hormonal changes that make physiologic cysts come and go during your reproductive years are not working anymore after menopause. The only thing that a repeat ultrasound will show is whether or not it is growing. If it is, it may be a tumor and should be removed. If it is NOT growing, it may be a physiologic cyst that you carried into menopause that never went away and never will. It's kind of frozen in time. A safe plan would be to discuss with your physician how many more ultrasounds and how often they should be done. This way, surgery can often be avoided.

Cysts between 5 and 10 cm are in a grey area as to the best plan in the postmenopausal years. The risk of cancer in these situations is about 1% if the cyst is "simple" and over 7.5cm in size. If the cyst has some solid parts, then the risk of cancer jumps to about 4%. That is still only 4 out of a 100, but you get the message. Be careful and discuss the risk compared to benefit of treatment with your doctor(s).

If you are postmenopausal, have a simple cyst of 5cm or less, have a normal CA125 level and there is no history of cancer in the immediate family (sisters, mom and aunts mainly), then the risk is lower than 1% and it may be reasonable to keep doing ultrasounds to make sure there is no growth. This is a situation where you have to work closely with your doctor, but in many cases a surgery can be avoided safely. If there is a question, see a gynecologic oncologist for a second opinion.

(6) If a benign appearing ovarian mass is found on ultrasound during your reproductive years that your doctor does NOT think is a physiologic or functional

cyst, surgery is usually recommended. The type of surgery is called a cystectomy (removal of the cystic mass only), not an oophorectomy (removal of the entire ovary) in most cases. This can often be done through a laparoscope (band-aid surgery) where you have surgery under general anesthesia, but using only three to four small incisions rather than through a bigger incision (laparotomy). A more advanced version of this is robotically assisted laparoscopic surgery which we cover later in depth in it's own book chapter.

If a cystic ovarian mass is considered possibly cancerous (based on how it looks on ultrasound and other factors, like your family history of cancer), then one of your surgeons should be a gynecologic oncologist. A gynecologic oncologist should also be consulted if you have had multiple surgeries, if there is even a remote chance that it could be cancer or if there is a strong suspicion of advanced endometriosis. In these situations, due to intense scarring and possible involvement of adjacent organs like the bladder and bowel, a surgeon who has a greater skillset than a general gynecologist may be very helpful for safe surgery. Again, that surgeon is a gynecologic oncologist.

One final note about treatment planning and accuracy of determining physiologic cysts vs benign tumors vs cancerous tumors. We are moving into a molecular age and tests for cancer are becoming extremely sensitive. However, the problem is that some are even too sensitive and raise the red flag of a possible cancer diagnosis inaccurately. These tests, largely based on circulating tumor DNA (ctDNA) are going to improve in accuracy over the upcoming years. If you are offered such a test, keep in mind that they are not ready for prime time yet and can be very misleading, not to mention anxiety producing if positive.

Fallopian Tube "Cysts" and Para-Ovarian Cysts

Paraovarian cysts are cysts which come from tissues near and around the ovaries, like the peritoneum (internal skin lining that we have which covers all of our internal organs). They are usually very small and usually do not cause problems. Even though they are not "tumors", they tend to stay and slowly grow over years. When found during an ultrasound they have the same characteristics as ovarian cysts, are usually simple (meaning no internal solid parts) and usually do not go away unless they rupture. That can cause temporary pain, just like an ovarian cyst rupture can. On the other hand they are usually extremely slow growing. The problem is that if they get a little larger, like greater than 3 cm or so, they can cause pain by undergoing twisting (torsion) just like an ovarian cyst. So, whether or not to remove these surgically depends on a lot of factors that you should discuss with your doctor. I just wanted you to be aware that these exist, but are usually innocent bystanders. They are rarely the cause of chronic cyst forming pain.

One other "cyst" that might be found on ultrasound or because you have pain is an enlargement of the Fallopian tube itself. This is called a "hydro-salpinx" and means the tube was somehow scarred (e.g. infection or endometriosis) and sealed off its open end. When that happens, the tube can fill up with fluid and look like a cyst on ultrasound. Usually the radiologist can tell it apart from an ovarian cyst because it looks more oblong or sausage-shaped. These do not go away on their own, and medical or natural alternatives will not make these disappear, regardless of what you do. So, whether or not to consider surgery depends upon a discussion with your trusted doctor about risks and benefits. The decision will largely depend upon whether or not it is causing you enough pain to go through a surgery to remove the tubes.

Tumors of the Ovary

Ovarian tumors are *very* different from ovarian physiologic cysts, but can look like cysts. Tumors are growths, due to piling up or overgrowth of benign or malignant cells. They will *never* go away on their own and if they are cancerous they can be life-threatening. Let's cover the most common types and some of the dangers of a missed diagnosis.

DERMOID CYSTS

A dermoid "cyst" is actually a tumor also known as a benign cystic teratoma or mature teratoma. Teratoma literally means "monsterous growth", and is called that because it may contain all sorts of tissues like glands, hair, bone, skin, hair and even teeth.

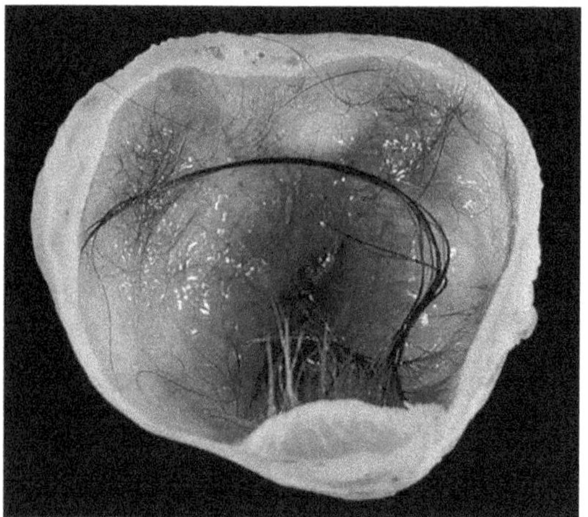

Figure 7: Dermoid Cyst (Source: Wikimedia, Ed Uthman MD, public domain)

Dermoids are very common during the reproductive years, but can occur from infancy and into the menopausal years. In fact, about one third of all benign (non cancer) tumors of the ovary found during the reproductive years are dermoid cysts. After menopause, this drops to about 20% of all benign tumors in that age range. There is a malignant type of dermoid, called an immature teratoma, but these are rare. Even more rare, mainly in women over 40, about 1% of benign dermoids can undergo something called malignant degeneration. In other words, part of the dermoid becomes malignant or cancerous over time.

Dermoid cysts can be single, multiple, on one or both ovaries, as tiny as a few millimeters or as large as 25-30 cm. However, it is unusual for them to be larger than 10cm, and they are visibly found on only one ovary almost 90% of the time. Microscopically they may be present in both ovaries but may not grow, or grow very slowly over many years.

In an ultrasound picture, dermoids can look pretty simple (single ballon sac-like and fluid filled) but the radiologist can usually see that the fluid inside is pretty thick. In fact, when they are removed surgically, the fluid is thick and creamy and called "sebaceous". The pathologist will often find hair balls and teeth, among other things in these little monsters.

So, how do these little monsters grow? From all of the research it looks like these start growing in the ovaries when you are still a developing baby inside your mother. Without getting into too much science and genetics, they arise from what are called "toti-potential stem cells" or very early egg cells in the ovary which can literally develop into any type of cell. This is why you find all different types of tissues in dermoids like hair, teeth, glands, muscle, nerves, cartilage and more. Again, toti-potential means these cells can literally turn into anything, and they do…inside the dermoid cyst.

About half of the time dermoids do not cause any symptoms at all and may be found during a routine pelvic examination or ultrasound. When they cause symptoms, they are usually the same as any other cystic mass in the pelvis can cause. They may cause pressure, achy pain, torsion and severe pain, and they may rupture and bleed.

Literally any type of tissue can grow inside a dermoid. In fact, in about 10% of dermoids, the pathologist can find thyroid tissue. When most of the tissue in there is thyroid type, the dermoid gets a special name: Struma Ovarii. Why is this important? Because in about 5% of these situations the thyroid hormones can be released in very large amounts leading to hyperthyroidism and thyrotoxicosis. Symptoms of these rare situations may be the same as one with overactive thyroid and include rapid unintentional weight loss despite a normal appetite, nervousness, restlessness, heat intolerance, fatigue, increased sweating, and menstrual irregularities, in some combination.

Abnormal intestinal or lung tissue can also grow inside a dermoid and cause strange symptoms. This is called a carcinoid tumor. The strange symptoms can include skin flushing, facial skin spider veins on the nose, frequent diarrhea, difficult breathing that is asthma-like and wheezing. These are very rare, but they do happen.

About 1% of all dermoids rupture at some point, spilling their thick irritating sebaceous fluid in the pelvis. This happens a little more frequently during pregnancy, possibly because the growing uterus puts more pressure on the dermoid, causing it to rupture or leak. The sebaceous fluid can be very irritating inside, causing severe pain, and sometimes requires emergency surgery to wash it out. Most of the time there is a slow leak rather than a rupture. But this can still lead to a severe reaction of your internal skin-like lining (peritoneum), causing peritonitis or inflammation. Peritonitis, in turn, causes pain. In some cases the scarring can be so severe that it can look like cancer and/or cause a kink in the intestine, not allowing food to go through. This is called a bowel obstruction and often requires surgery to straighten things out. If the leak or rupture occurs during pregnancy, the irritation to the uterus can cause preterm labor.

Finally, as can happen with any cyst, twisting (torsion) of the supporting ligaments and blood vessels can also occur with dermoid cysts. Dermoids are "heavy" because of the all the tissues in them, so it actually happens more frequently than with other cysts (up to 10% of the time). So, one in ten women with a dermoid can expect emergency surgery at some point in time for torsion, unless the dermoid is removed before this happens.

So, when should treatment be sought? The good news is that it can take years for these to grow. Dermoids only grow about 1 or 2mm per year. After the dermoid cyst is felt by your doctor and the ultrasound pretty much confirms it, it could take a while before it causes problems. In the old days, or if ultrasound is not available, a plain X-ray of the pelvic area can show the bone and teeth that can be found in many dermoids. If it is still uncertain after the ultrasound, an MRI may be helpful.

How should these be treated? Eventually, surgery will be required because dermoid cysts will never go away and will continue to grow. The good news is that this can usually be done by laparoscopy or robotic surgery (band-aid surgery). Often, only the cyst can be removed and not the whole ovary. When the cysts get to be around 10cm or so, the chances of a leak during removal of the cyst increases. For that reason, for larger dermoid tumors, many doctors prefer to remove them through an open incision (laparotomy). This largely depends on the surgeon's skill and experience but you should always ask about a minimally invasive (band-aid) surgery approach. Even larger ones can be put inside a bag to reduce spill of the fluid and then be removed using minimally invasive surgery, through a small incision.

So how does one decide if it is time to do surgery? If your doctor thinks you have a dermoid, and you already have symptoms due to pressure, torsion or possible leak, the time is now. Especially with leaking fluid, scars continue to form and the surgery becomes tougher and tougher to perform safely without injuring nearby organs and intestines. Also, if the dermoid is between 5 and 10cm and you are pregnant, your doctor may recommend removing it to avoid rupture and pre-term labor. This is something you need to discuss with your Ob-Gyn physician in detail. There are risks and benefits to waiting or to going ahead with the surgery. The best time for surgery during pregnancy is during the second trimester for multiple medical reasons, including least risk of losing the baby.

If you have no symptoms, are not pregnant, and the dermoid cyst is less than 5cm or so, it may be reasonable to wait. However, remember that these cysts tend to twist (torsion) and cause severe pain more than other cysts and that they can leak or rupture that irritating pain-producing sebaceous fluid at any time. So, it's sort of like a ticking time bomb inside of you because it will simply continue to grow until something happens. Remember, dermoids will not go away on their own and won't get smaller unless they leak or rupture. So, it may be better to get it over with while it is relatively easy to do through minimally invasive surgery.

There is one more thing that should be part of your decision-making. Those little monster dermoids tend to grow back, because microscopic ones may not be seen during surgery and therefore not removed. So, especially if you are through with childbearing and especially if there are already a number of dermoids growing in the ovary (not just one), you might want to talk with your doctor about taking the whole ovary out to prevent having to go through surgery multiple times. Usually, the other ovary can be left behind because dermoids tend to be in both ovaries only 10-15% of the time. Again, this is a risk vs. benefit discussion that you have to have with a trusted physician. The treatment strategy is generally the same, from the US to China and everywhere in between.

OTHER CYSTIC OVARIAN TUMORS

Cystic teratomas or dermoids are the most common benign tumor of the ovary, but there are many others. I won't get into the rare ones, because it is not the focus of this book, but there are a few others which deserve being mentioned. These can also look like cysts on ultrasound, but may also have some solid parts. Most are benign and not cancerous. These are the cystadenomas (mucinous or serous) and cystadenofibromas. Figure 8 shows one type of these cystic tumors. To an expert pathologist, they will each look a little different, but for you the main thing is to appreciate that there are "cystic" or hollow areas in all of these tumors. There may be one cystic area, or many clustered together. On an ultrasound, it may look like a bunch of regular physiologic cysts, but they are way different because they are tumors and not cysts. As mentioned, tumors may be benign or malignant. Malignant ones (cancer) tend to grow much faster, can spread to other parts of your body (metastasize) and can kill you. With rare exception, benign ovarian tumors do not spread to other parts of the body, but will continue to grow and can cause all of the problems we already discussed in terms of pain, torsion, rupture and bleeding. Eventually, surgery is necessary to remove these. The urgency for surgery depends upon multiple factors that make it more likely that the tumor is actually a cancer. This might be family history of cancer, positive genetic testing, how ugly it looks on ultrasound, blood tests and more.

One more thing before we touch on cancer. Sometimes a tumor can be "borderline" or "low malignant potential". This means that it may look ugly under the microscope but rarely spreads to other areas, does not require additional treatment like chemo and is usually not life threatening.

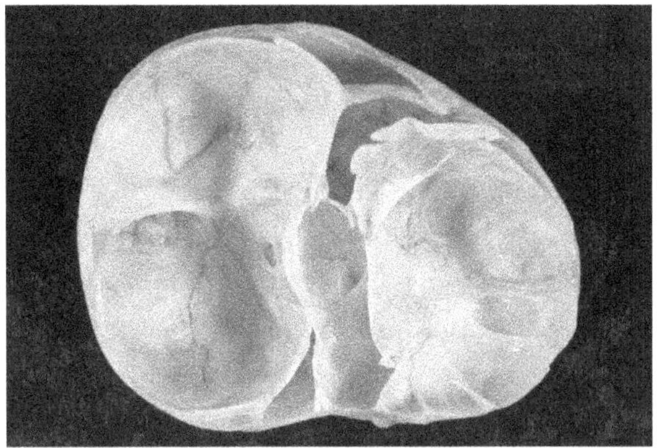

Figure 8: Mucinous Cystadenoma (Source: Wikimedia, Ed Uthman MD, public domain)

OVARIAN CANCER

Cancer, or malignant tumors of the ovary, are rarely caught early and can threaten your life. Over 75% of the time ovarian cancer is diagnosed in late stages when it has already spread. Worse, there are no good screening tools to detect early ovarian cancer.

If you don't have a family history of breast or ovarian cancer then the lifetime risk of developing this potentially lethal disease is about 2%. That seems low but when it happens it is very difficult to treat. So, attention to health, prevention and early diagnosis when possible is the goal. If you have a genetic mutation (BRCA1, BRCA2 and others) your risk goes up markedly and means at some point in life you may want to have your ovaries removed before they become cancerous. This is what happened to Angelina Jolie.

Certainly if you have a genetic mutation and a mass is found on your ovary, while this does not automatically mean it is cancer, there is urgency to be fully evaluated by the right doctor. That right doctor is a gynecologic oncologist.

In fact, there are different types of ovarian cancer. If an ovarian mass is suspicious for cancer, in order to determine the best treatment plan, a gynecologic oncologist will order blood tests called "tumor markers". CA-125 is only one of these.

Which ones are ordered depends largely on age. The younger you are, the more the cancer may be a special kind called germ cell or stromal cancer. For those the tumor markers are usually called alpha-feto protein (AFP), lactate dehydrogenase (LDH), beta-HCG (the pregnancy hormone), and inhibin A and B. The older you are, the more it is likely an epithelial ovarian cancer for which CA-125, CEA and CA 19-9 are the more commonly checked markers. An OVA-1, as discussed above, may also be checked as it is a combination of markers and provides a general "risk of malignancy" range to help determine which surgeons should be involved. In other words, whether or not a gynecologic oncologist should be involved in your surgery is partly signaled by results of these tumor markers. The more they are elevated, the more you should have an expert cancer surgeon in your corner.

Ovarian cancer or a mass or cyst on the ovary that is suspicious for ovarian cancer is usually treated surgically by removal. Whether or not it is safe to just remove the cystic mass or not depends on the exact circumstances. But removal of the mass or removal of the ovary is the first step. If cancer is diagnosed, usually by rapid analysis in the operating room called a "frozen section", then additional biopsies are performed to make sure the cancer has not spread. Sometimes no additional treatment, like chemo, is required. But this depends on what the cancer looks like under the microscope and what the additional biopsies show.

Ovarian cancer surgery often continues to be done through a big incision called a laparotomy, which takes months to heal. More and more surgeons are becoming capable of minimally invasive surgery, even when cancer is present. A minimally invasive approach is not always possible. However, when it is, it significantly speeds up recovery and gets you to the next phase of any additional required treatment as soon as possible. More on minimally invasive surgery later in this book, focusing specifically on robotic surgery for cancer or ovarian masses suspicious for cancer.

Talking With Your Doctor(s)

Here are some tips if your doctor suspects an ovarian tumor, rather than a cyst. Your doctor will be going through a process of what is called "differential diagnosis" in their head, using what they know, what they researched for your specific case and all the specific findings and symptoms you have, including examination and scans. This means, they try to put it all together and decide what it is most likely to be in their professional opinion. In some centers, these combined factors are plugged into a computer model and artificial intelligence (AI) spits out the likely risk of cancer. But in most centers, it is still mainly the doctor making a clinical decision based on this information.

Hopefully, especially using the information in this book, you have been able to find a trusted doctor with whom you can discuss the options in detail. If you aren't sure how much thought they have put in to your case, or what experience they have, do yourself a favor. ASK THEM!! Point blank. It's your body and you have the right to know why a recommendation is being made and on what basis. If you are under the care of someone who wants to operate on you and is not explaining WHY you need surgery in a way that you can understand, there is only one thing to do…RUN! Find someone you trust who can explain it to you. In all fairness, please understand that they may be right. Also, "doctor-shopping" is never a good idea because it can get very confusing. But a reasonable discussion with a doctor that you can connect with, in terms that you can understand, prior to going to surgery is prudent.

Likewise, if you are being asked to "wait it out," then ask what the risks are in YOUR particular situation. Be proactive. It's your body we're talking about here. You absolutely positively need to establish a doctor-patient relationship that works for you. Learn and understand the basics in this book, then incorporate information about your specific situation which you should be getting from your doctor.

What kind of a doctor you have, meaning what specialty, can also make a difference. At the very least, if you have ovarian cysts you should see a gynecologist. Regardless of what other practitioners are involved, a gynecologist can help order the right tests and advise you about all of the mainstream medical and surgical options. I can't emphasize enough how important it is to try to get the right diagnosis before starting on any kind of treatment plan, mainstream or natural/holistic.

If there is ANY suspicion at all that the "cyst" may be cancerous, you would really do yourself a HUGE favor by seeing a gynecologic oncologist for a second opinion. Trust me. It could save your life, and gynecologic oncologists are the LEAST likely to do surgery if it is really not necessary. Why? Because they are extremely used to seeing the ugly cysts that are most likely to be cancerous and are pretty darned familiar with what that looks like.

If you feel that all doctors are crooks and/or money grubbing, are in cahoots with a nefarious government FDA conspiracy to keep you away from a healthy non-surgical answer, and will sell you out for a buck, I can't change your mind or help you. On the other hand, if you find yourself under the care of someone that you are developing a mature doctor-patient professional relationship with, the thoughts above apply.

With regard to gynecologic oncologists specifically, these are docs who are used to seeing the whole range of simple to horrific, including cancer. If it is a simple cyst you probably don't need a gynecologic oncologist's opinion. But if it is possible cancer, find one and get that second opinion.

Prevention

There are a number of ways to prevent physiologic or functional ovarian cysts from forming, or at least reducing the chances that they will. The mainstream Western medicine way to do this is by using "the pill" or oral contraceptives. There are quite a few types out there and almost all are considered "low dose".

Even if this may be considered a "safe" prevention for ovarian physiologic or functional cysts, there are some very important things you should know. First of all, every medication has some side effects. These can be slightly different between the different types of oral contraceptives and you should work with your doctor in deciding which one is best for you. Oral contraceptives do vary in the type and amount of synthetic estrogen and progestin they contain, and there are quite a few variations.

If you are looking for a more natural version, unfortunately, at this time there are no bio-identical fully "natural" oral contraceptive pills to even consider in the United States. Almost all of the synthetic hormone oral contraceptives will increase the level of a protein in your blood called "sex hormone binding globulin." This protein, when it is increased can bind or "hold on to" testosterone that is normally produced in your body and make it unavailable to exert its normal effects. The effect you may notice is decreased sex drive. Also, since the pill can reduce Vitamins C and B6 in your body, this can affect some of the normal chemicals in your brain called neurotransmitters. When these go out of whack, you might feel depressed. So, consider supplementing your diet with Vitamins C and B6 if you are on an oral contraceptive or "the pill."

More importantly, you should not be taking oral contraceptive pills if you:

1. Smoke and are over the age of 35

2. Have high blood pressure which is out of control*
3. Have diabetes which is out of control*
4. Have heart disease*
5. Have had a heart attack or stroke
6. Have a history of blood clots in your veins or lungs
7. Get chest pains or "angina"
8. Have or are at risk for cancer of the breast, uterus, or cervix
9. Have active liver disease
10. Have had liver tumors (cancerous or noncancerous)
11. Have had jaundice (yellowing of the skin and whites of the eyes) during pregnancy
12. Have any abnormal vaginal bleeding that has not been checked out
13. Are pregnant or think you might be
14. Have an allergy or hypersensitivity reactions to oral contraceptives
15. Have kidney disease
16. Have adrenal insufficiency (adrenals are organs near your kidneys)
17. Have severe headaches
18. Have had major surgery and are not able to move around very much

* If you have diabetes or blood pressure problems, birth control pills are not the best idea for you, but in some cases it is better than the problems you might face if you get pregnant. So, discuss this with your trusted doctor(s).

Finally, to round out a scary long list, if you are taking any other prescription medications or herbals/supplements, talk with your doctor and/or pharmacist about possible incompatibility or cross-reaction with oral contraceptives.

The good news is this. If you do not have any of the above, MANY scientific research studies over many years have been done which document that oral contraceptives are really very safe to take. In fact, other than staying pregnant your whole life (multiple back to back pregnancies), taking oral contraceptives is the only PROVEN means by which to actually REDUCE the risk of ovarian cancer, short of removing the ovaries. One of the theories is based on less ovulation which means less trauma to the ovary, which means less risk of something going wrong with the healing process and turning into cancer.

So, even though oral contraceptives may not be a perfect solution, and they are certainly not a "natural" solution, they may save you a lot of pain and concern by preventing physiologic cyst formation and prevent ovarian cancer. You might at least want to consider this for a short time to get rid of repetitive pain from multiple cysts while you decide upon other strategies for prevention.

Alternative and Complementary Options

First, let's get a few definitions straight. Alternative treatment usually means using a natural substance or technique INSTEAD of standard Western medical recommendations. This includes but is not limited to nutritional dietary alteration, herbals, supplements, Traditional Chinese and Ayurvedic solutions, psychosocial mind-body strategies and physical manipulation. If you decide to approach treatment this way, you should seek licensed practitioners who have experience in treating such conditions and preferably who cooperate with Western allopathic doctors. With a licensed practitioner, who has credentials from a reputable school, at least you have some idea as to the credentials, capabilities and track record of your provider. There are certainly alternative practitioners around the world who have a verifiable track record of experience and results, but it may be more difficult to find this out. Your first goal should be *not* to get into the hands of someone who might harm you or rip you off. Ask questions. 'Nuff said.

Complementary or integrative solutions mean using methods which are used TOGETHER with standard Western approaches to improve the chances of success or to help your symptoms of pain, bleeding, stress, anxiety and so forth. There is obviously some room for overlap between East and West philosophies towards seeking a comprehensive holistic approach, otherwise known as integrative medicine.

A word about "evidence" and "proof." Please remember that "hope" is not a good strategy for anything. You probably want some idea of what the chances are that something will actually work rather than simply hoping that it will because someone said so. Miracles abound, but you would probably agree that they usually occur less frequently than someone winning the lottery. So, while that might happen to you, here is a breakdown of what you might want to look out for.

Everything that is written in books, scientific papers, testimonials and the internet is NOT the same in terms of validity. The strongest evidence of proof that something will work is based on something called "prospective randomized clinical trials". This means that a group of scientists, doctors and statisticians got together and designed a study to compare one treatment to another. This type of study is designed to *reliably* prove or disprove something. Half of the patients get one treatment and the other half get another. Who gets what is based on a computerized version of a coin toss: "heads or tails." The study is done over months to years and the results are rigorously analyzed to see if the conclusions are valid or not. This is the gold standard for comparing very specific treatments like drug A vs. drug B. However, when looking at broader treatments like a combination of herbs or a dietary modification, these kinds of studies are not ideal to determine whether or not the treatment worked. So this means that this "gold standard" of scientific evidence can't be readily applied to all things.

In some cases it is not practical to design a randomized clinical trial because it would take a zillion patients to reliably prove that something works better than the other option. So the next best set of tools include large "non-randomized prospective reviews", "case controlled" and "cohort" epidemiologic studies. There are pretty good but there are a lot of statistical problems and "biases" introduced which may mask the truth.

The next level is "retrospective reviews" and "case reports" or "case series" which describe what happened in a situation where a good result was observed. The biases here are even greater and this is akin to basic "testimonials." This means that if the information was collected accurately, completely and truthfully, it is possible that the treatment might work. But this is based on a small sample of results. In some cases it is only ONE person's results. It MAY work, but based on this level of evidence it is said to be "unproven". Sometimes if the results are plausible (i.e. some reasonable scientific explanation for the result exists), particularly if there is laboratory (e.g. petri dish) and animal research proof, it is certainly something that may be "proven" in the future. In other words, it may work.

It's important to realize that absence of proof that something works or not is not the only important thing. There is also a question of *harm*. Is it possible that something worked for one individual, but the next one will drop dead from side effects and complications? The answer is always YES until better research information, usually through clinical trials, is available. Suffice it to say that testimonials are very weak evidence that something works. It does not mean it will not work. It just means it is very very sketchy if there is no better evidence to support the claims made.

Stay smart, be safe, and don't do anything without looking at the details of what you are putting into yourself first. Get several opinions if you are not sure. Read about it, paying attention to the credibility of the source. Is there research being quoted or is it all just anecdotal testimonials?

Having said all that, due to multiple reasons including lack of funds, there has been very little quality research done in alternative and integrative healthcare. This does not mean that any given practice or treatment does not work. It simply means that it is unproven and may not be safe. Another problem is that supplements and herbals are not subject to rigorous quality control. So be cautious. The newest laws call for "good manufacturing practices" or GMPs. At the very least, whenever you buy supplements and herbals, make sure you buy from a manufacturing laboratory that is certified in this area.

One last comment about evidence. Almost *anyone* can write a book these days. For sure anyone with a computer can blog on a website. Actually, you don't even need a computer. You can find one in an internet café. So just because it is there does not mean the information contained in a blog or website is accurate.

Books also get old very quickly. So, even though there are classic, even ancient, healthcare books out there, in general the art and science of health care are both advancing very rapidly. You should be looking at whether or not the article or book you are reading is quoting recent information, like recent research publications. These days alternative and complementary remedies are finding their way into mainstream journals as well as their own dedicated journals. At the very least it is fresh information that the journal board has reviewed and judged to be reasonable for publication based on quality criteria. These criteria are not perfect, but they are FAR better than nothing, which is what you find on many websites in general.

One last warning or caveat. Remember that there are unscrupulous individuals out there that are willing to market literally ANYTHING to you for one reason. Money. Please beware and don't get caught up in the hype. Learn first, and then decide.

Natural Prevention Strategies

Are there alternatives to birth control pills for physiologic cyst formation? Yes, there are, but the evidence for their effectiveness may not be as good and details of what works better than the next thing are hard, or impossible, to come by. So, you take a risk that these treatments may not work, and it is hard to recommend which one(s) to start with. But we have looked into what might be the best shot you have at deciding where to start.

This next point is VERY important. In making your decisions you might also want to pay attention to whether or not there is some kind of evidence or proof that you won't be harmed by what you're taking. Re-read the section above about what level of proof you should be looking for. Having said that, there are plenty of cultures around the world where there are no synthetic hormone oral contraceptives and women have been using natural techniques for years. Some of these, like dietary and nutritional changes are very unlikely to harm you and have a great chance of helping you. On the other hand, when you get into specific herbals and supplements just pay attention to what you are doing. Are you sure that it is safe, based on the evidence that you read or from factual and verifiable information your practitioner tells you about? Is taking a higher dose safe? OK, let's start in with what you can do…starting with what is at least suggested to be most effective and so on, down the list.

NUTRITION AND DIET

Treating and preventing ovarian cysts using healthy diets and exercise to lose weight are mainly intended for those women with PCOS. You have seen how there are different cysts and they form due to different reasons under different influences. But, as noted before, there may be some biochemical overlap between the condition of PCOS and physiologic cyst formation with no other findings or symptoms. Because of this, a good nutrition and supplement strategy will not hurt and may very well help anyone forming physiologic cysts, PCOS or not. Women with PCOS definitely have bigger and broader problems associated with being overweight and diabetes. So, an anti-diabetic diet and exercise works to improve androgen profile and influence cyst formation in this way. If you are in this situation, please consult a nutrition practitioner about an appropriate diet designed for you. In general, such a diet includes an increase in fiber intake and a decrease in refined carbohydrates (simple sugars), as well as a decrease in trans- and saturated fats and an increase in omega-3 and omega-9 fatty acids (fish oil). In general, the percent fat in your diet should be less that 30%. However, if it is only plant fats, like avocado, then a higher % is fine. It is also generally helpful to eat foods that are anti-inflammatory, including fiber, omega-3 fatty acids, vitamin E, and some red wine.

As far as scientific proof regarding how well supplements work, here are a few important ones. A study from Germany found that Vitamin D can affect insulin resistance and diabetes and thus have an impact on PCOS indirectly.

Another study showed that there is definitely something wrong with Vitamin D and Calcium metabolism in women with PCOS, which was partly reversed when Vitamin D and Calcium supplementation was started.

Many natural therapy gurus recommend Vitamin A in ovarian cyst and PCOS treatment. There are no studies which show a benefit and some reports suggest *harm*. In other words, use of Vitamin A and its related carotenoids can *cause* someone to develop or perhaps accelerate development of PCOS. Actually, there is scientific evidence that this can happen because of how Vitamin A and retinoids affect insulin resistance and Vitamin A or retinoid receptors on the ovaries. So, this is a great example of how a "natural therapy" can harm you and be useless.

Summary of Cyst Preventing Dietary Guidelines:

- Grab a book on nutrition and healthy diets and put together a diet that works for you including the following:
    - No more than 30% fat. Again, this can be a little higher percentage if it is only plant fats. (this influences steroid hormone production)
    - Whole grain complex carbohydrates (carbs)

  - NO simple sugars including sucrose (table sugar) and even minimize fructose (from fruit)
  - Anti-oxidant and anti-inflammatory foods (tomatoes, greens, fish)
    - Tip: You can't really go wrong with the Mediterranean Diet, which even includes a little wine.
    - Tip: Generally, the healthiest anti-disease diet is a whole food plant-based diet. "Based" is the key word, because that is the main food you eat, to which you can add fish and other lean animal protein if you so choose, in moderation.
- Eliminate caffeine (stressor) and limit alcohol (simple sugar)
- Supplements to consider adding:
  - Vitamin B-6 (especially if on birth control pills), and B-complex in general
  - Vitamin C
  - Vitamin D (you can ask for a blood test to determine if you are taking enough)
  - Vitamin E
  - Omega-3 and Omega-9 Essential Fatty Acids

Some have recommended adding Zinc and Selenium, but scientific studies have been done which show no difference in Zinc levels between women with no cysts, benign cysts and ovarian tumors. Regarding Selenium, there is no human data but in cows, where they are also concerned about fertility for breeding, those with higher Selenium levels had a *higher* chance of having ovarian cysts.

HERBAL REMEDIES

An herbal derivative that is being used for many conditions as an anti-inflammatory and pain relief method is CBD oil. CBD is a cannabis compound (cannabinoid) and CBD oil is an extract combined with a carrier oil. While marijuana has become legalized in more and more places, it is the THC (tetrahydrocannabinol) that is the psychoactive component that makes someone "stoned" and is the reason for legality issues. Pure CBD on the other hand does not contain THC (mixtures definitely exist for a combined anti-inflammatory and psychoactive calming effect), and therefore is legal in most areas. How CBD works is very complex but may be partly external, as an anti-inflammatory, and partly internal by interfacing with the endo-cannabinoid system that exists naturally in people. So, for cysts and endometriosis, there is reason to consider this as a better alternative to narcotics or non-narcotic medications that can wreak havoc on your stomach lining.

Herbs that have been recommended for physiologic cyst prevention, with little or no published proof are: black cohosh, St.John's wort, burdock, dandelion, mullein, red raspberry, nettles, yarrow, vitex and Siberian ginseng. Kava and valerian root have also been recommended as a way to de-stress and one can use the mind-body or psychoneuroimmunology connection to prevent cysts, which we write about later in this book. Chinese herbs include astragalus, ginger, dong quai, cinnamon, rehmannia root, and scrophularia root. It is unclear what science would be used to come up with a tailored combination and which combinations would work the best, but these are the ones individually recommended the ***most***, based on many sources and folklore. We'll get into specific formulations and combinations published in the Traditional Chinese Medicine scientific literature in a bit. In general, taking too many things at once is a very bad idea because you have no idea what is working and what is not, and you can interfere with prescription medications. In some cases, these interactions can be severe and potentially fatal.

While most herbs and supplements are probably safe to take in general, everyone is different. Your metabolism is not exactly the same as the person next to you and anything that is taken in excess can cause problems. The problem is that herbs and supplements are made by a lot of different companies who may or may not be ethical and may or may not have good manufacturing practices. So, you may not be getting what it says your getting on the bottle or box. My advice to you is to stick to "name brands" or do some research with your trusted healthcare practitioner before you buy. There are different "no-name" brands all over the world, making it difficult to make recommendations for everyone.

Even if you take herbs and supplements responsibly, you should also know that there are possible complications and side effects, just like prescription medicines. Here are some of the more important things to watch out for, especially if you might be facing surgery or are taking prescription medications. Remember, talk with your doctor about any herbals you might be taking. This is just a brief introduction to what you should be thinking whenever you start taking something new. Check everything out BEFORE you run into problems, especially if surgery to remove a cystic tumor is a possibility.

Echinacea

Echinacea is very commonly used as an immune stimulant to prevent and treat early "colds." But when used longer than 8 weeks, it can actually suppress your immune system. This could mean an easier chance of catching one of those mean bugs in the hospital while you're trying to recover from surgery, and can also interfere with wound healing.

Echinacea can affect your liver, especially if you already have liver problems or are taking medications which affect your liver. When combined with surgical anesthesia medications, liver failure can result. For all these reasons, even a simple surgery can turn into a disaster just by taking this simple herbal medication. To reduce these complication risks, Echinacea should be discontinued at least several weeks before surgery.

Ephedra

Ephedra, widely used as a weight-loss supplement until it was banned in 2003, can increase blood pressure and heart rate. Fatal and near fatal events related to this were the reason it was banned. However, personal stockpiles are still out there and are doubly dangerous around the time of surgery. If you are hoarding a pile of these pills, do yourself a favor. GET RID OF THEM! There are better ways to lose weight.

Ephedra, when used in combination with the common anesthesia gas Halothane, can lead to dangerous and life-threatening arrhythmias. In addition, other interaction with commonly used perioperative medications can lead to permanent heart damage and, in the worst case, coma. Ephedra, if you actually using it despite all the warnings, should be discontinued at least 24 hours before surgery.

Garlic

Garlic is widely used to lower cholesterol, decrease the risk of blood clots and reduce blood pressure. The problem is that reduction in blood clot risk is accomplished by an effect on platelets, something you need to clot properly during and after surgery. So, while it is doing its job it can lead to fatal uncontrolled bleeding. Stop using Garlic at least 7 to 10 days prior to surgery.

Ginko

Ginko has long been used to improve memory, reduce atherosclerosis, treat erectile dysfunction, among other uses. There are several biochemical reasons for its effectiveness, one of which is inhibition of platelet function. Again, platelets are needed to help with blood clotting. Major complications and deaths have been reported. It is best to stop using Ginko at least 36 hours before surgery.

Ginseng

Ginseng has multiple species which are used for medicinal treatment. The most commonly used are Asian and American Ginseng. A number of these ginsenosides have been labeled "adaptogens" because of their ability to help protect the body against stress and restore homeostasis (internal systems order). There is concern about reversible and irreversible effects on platelets, which can cause bleeding disasters. In addition, ginsenosides can lower blood glucose. Since there are multiple ginsenosides, a recommendation about when to stop them before surgery is difficult to make. However, at least a week is prudent.

Kava

Kava, derived from the pepper plant Piper methysticum, is often used as a sedative and anxiety reducing agent. Since multiple sedatives are used around the time of surgery, additional sedation and interaction with these medications has led to coma. Kava should be discontinued at least a day or two before surgery.

St. John's Wort

St John's Wort, or Hypericum perforatum, is used by many for mild to moderate depression. It works by interfering with chemicals called neurotransmitters in your brain. It can also significantly increase the metabolism of many medications used around the time of surgery, reducing their effectiveness. These medications include lidocaine, midazolam hydrochloride, calcium channel blockers, serotonin receptor antagonists, steroids, digoxin and warfarin. While you many not be familiar with all or most of these, they are commonly used in routine care or for management of complications. St John's Wort should be discontinued at least five days prior to surgery.

Valerian

Valerian is a sedative herbal, used in the treatment of insomnia. The more you take, the greater the effect. It also multiplies the effect of other sedatives routinely used around the time of surgery. Valerian withdrawal can be severe and further complicate surgical recovery. It is best to slowly reduce the dose of valerian if you have been taking it for a while to avoid withdrawal. If that is not possible because the surgery date is near, it may be best to continue valerian use and manage withdrawal as needed.

Clearly, it is best to discuss use of herbal medications with your surgeon as soon as possible. Even the most innocent commonly used herbs can cause major problems. So, here's a tip: Keep a running list of all medications that you take, prescription and natural. It is always a good idea, and in the event of surgery (especially emergency surgery for a ruptured bleeding cyst) you will run a lower risk of forgetting something critical.

Traditional Chinese Medicine Herbal Combination Therapy

Modern variations and scientific documentation of Traditional Chinese Medicine (TCM) remedies really only started coming to Western attention in the 1980's when we started seeing publications from journals like *Abstracts of Chinese Medicine* (1986) and *Traditional Chinese Medicine* (1981). The last one is published in English, by the way, so you can check it out and research it personally.

Of course, a lot of these remedies have been in print since the Inner Canon of the Yellow Emperor (Huangdi Neijing), from the 1st century BCE. Many would argue that it goes back 4000 years earlier than that! Wow, at first glance this is incredible and it is impressive that there are more than two thousands years of experience with remedies that supposedly work well. While modern TCM journals are publishing what might actually work, remember that the vast majority of these remedies have NOT been proven to work when carefully tested…at least not yet. So, while these remedies are something to explore, keep in mind that as recently as 150 years ago Radium was used to "treat" many conditions. Radium is a naturally occurring radioactive substance, but it can kill you (think Chernobyl). It didn't take much science, once we realized what it was, to figure out that this was a very bad idea. But without science pushing us forward to understand what is good or bad and why, we could still be in the dark ages in many ways. So, just because someone thought some remedy is a good idea, today or back in the Qing Dynasty, without scientific proof of safety and efficacy we should simply be careful. Having mentioned this important disclaimer, let's press on with what might be promising from the Chinese perspective.

In the Traditional Chinese Medicine (TCM) model, simple ovarian functional cysts are not considered to be very important by themselves. They are usually treated as part of other medical problems, like infertility in which hormonal imbalance and cyst formation is related to not being able to get pregnant.

Endometrioma/endometriosis and Polycystic Ovary Syndrome (PCOS) are treated very similarly in China compared to the USA, with the exception of herbals and acupuncture being added in many reports. These are far more complex diseases than simple functional or physiologic cysts and no one is effectively treating them with herbs alone, even in China or India. Before we cover herbals for simple cysts, you should know that modern TCM does not recommend treating benign tumors (like ovarian dermoid or cystadenoma) or cancer by herbals alone.

From a TCM perspective, fluid filled cysts on the ovary are really an accumulation of "phlegm" or "tan" as a sign of congestion, just like you might find in lung congestion during a bad cold. Why does it accumulate and stagnate in the ovary as phlegm? According to TCM teachings, it is because the kidney fails to "steam" the lower body's water upwards. To treat this, the water steaming function of the kidney is supported by cinnamon bark (rougui) and moisture regulation is supported by hoelen (fuling). This is an oversimplified explanation, and the rest of the theory can be found by studying yin/yang balance which also considers the right and left kidney as being different in function.

There are two main concoctions of ingredients: (1) Cinnamon and Hoelen [Gui Zhi Fu Ling Wan] and (2) Cinnamon and Rehmannia [Yang He Tang]. These formulas are adjusted for numerous issues which you would need to consult an experienced TCM practitioner about. However, here are the basic ingredients for these two formulas:

Cinnamon and Rehmannia Combination:

Chinese Name	English Name	Amount
shoudihuang	Rehmanni	30 grams
lujiaojiao	Antler gelatin	9 grams
rougui	Cinnamon bark	3 grams
paojiang	Roasted ginger	2 grams
baijiezi	sinapsis	6 grams
mahuang	Ma-huang	2 grams
gancao	licorice	3 grams

Cinammon and Hoelen Combination:

Chinese Name	English Name	Amount
Fu ling	(Hoelen) Poria	4 grams
Mu Dan Pi (Su)	Moutan	4 grams
Tao Ren	Persica	4 grams
Bai Shao (Shao yao)	Peony (white)	4 grams
Rou Gui (Gui zhi)	Cinnamon bark	4 grams

There are many variations of these formulas, and you can find them in your health food stores which carry herbals, but the above is the closest to the original ones as described in the Qing Dynasty in the 1700's. Turning our attention back to modern TCM, a limited number of studies have been published which indirectly tell us that Chinese herbal medications can affect the hormones which, in turn, affect cyst formation. This shows that there may be a scientific explanation for TCM herbal effect on ovarian cysts. However, we could find no direct published proof that they work in preventing functional or physiologic ovarian cysts. Consult your TCM practitioner for further details. However, again, I would like to ***strongly*** encourage you to work with a Western mainstream gynecologist as well so that you do not get into trouble with unproven therapy and miss something serious.

Let's move on to another possible way to attack your ovarian cyst problem.

ESTROGEN DOMINANCE AND BIO-IDENTICAL HORMONES

Ok, so here's the scoop on "natural" progesterone which is used by many women to "balance" their hormones. This is based on a theory of "estrogen dominance" made popular by the late Dr. Lee, which suggested that there is too much estrogen at any point in a woman's life and that the real problem was a relative deficiency in progesterone. What we know now is that women have normal progesterone levels during the reproductive years. However, due to environmental and lifestyle factors, there may indeed be relatively too much estrogen to keep a healthy balance. This can be from being overweight, knowingly or unknowingly taking estrogen or an estrogenic herbal or from xeno-estrogens, which arise from toxins in your environment. When hormonal balance falters, among other things, ovarian cysts form. But is there a way to truly "balance" your hormones by taking medications, herbals or anything else?

Those that suggest you can, prescribe bio-identical progesterone for the last part of your menstrual cycle. Bio-identical or "natural" progesterone is available in many forms, including a cream, which can applied to your skin as well as oral pills that you can swallow or put under your tongue. These are manufactured from Mexican yams and prepared by "compounding pharmacies". The problem is that no one is really regulating these pharmacies very well. So, as they say, "you take your chances". The creams can vary in strength by 10 to 20 times, which means you can overdose yourself. What does that mean? Other than health effects you may not see or feel immediately, you may gain a whole lot of weight because progesterone is "anabolic". It can also cause blood clots in your veins. Finally, we know that progesterone is a "mitogen" in the breast and uterus among other tissues and organs. What that means is that progesterone (natural or otherwise) stimulates cellular growth, which can become abnormal growth… even progressing to cancer. Most women will probably NOT get cancer from using progesterone. But you might grow your uterine fibroids, which are benign tumors that can cause pain! Remember, whenever you do something, there is a possible consequence. This is a big grey area in scientific research. So, buyer beware. You do not want to have too much estrogen, but you don't want too much progesterone either.

This part is worth repeating regardless of what you decide to do. At the very least listen to your trusted health practitioner regarding which compounding pharmacy is reliable and uses good manufacturing practices and ethics. Stay under the care of a licensed knowledgeable healthcare practitioner. Compounding pharmacies are not adequately regulated, so you literally have no idea what you might be getting. So before you beat the FDA up too badly, this safety issue is the dark side of inadequate regulations.

Many alternative practitioners propose that you measure progesterone levels in your saliva to see if therapy is working. While it is true that you can see changes in saliva levels, it is not clear what any given level means. No one knows what too much or too little is in terms of overall short or long-term effect on your body and it varies on an ongoing basis. No one can tell you that if the saliva level, or even a blood level, is at a certain point that you will or will not make uterine fibroids grow for example. The information is simply not worked out very well yet. So, please remember, anything you put inside your body can have consequences, whether it is "natural" or synthetic. Anything!

Let's look at it from another angle. Is there a way that we can reduce the amount of circulating estrogen and therefore "balance" hormones that way? Multiple studies show that circulating estrogen levels are higher in Western Europe and the USA than many other countries. For example, one study showed that estrogen among premenopausal Finnish women was 46% higher than that of Asian women. Another older study put it closer to 50% higher in those that are more meat eating compared to vegetarians.

A more recent Italian study showed that diet can make a world of difference in circulating estrogen levels. After six months, postmenopausal women who were placed on a Mediterranean diet reduced their estrogen levels by 40%.

Certain seaweeds, notably bladderwrack, can also reduce estrogen levels. An average estrogen lowering dose is about five grams, which is not hard to achieve. This can have an effect on "balancing" excess estrogen and reduce the risk of some cancers and endometriosis.

Insulin resistance and androgen bioavailability can also be reduced by diet and phytoestrogen (plant estrogen) supplementation. A healthy diet and exercise will increase sex hormone binding globulin (SHBG) and thus limit free or available estrogen by binding to it more. Diet and exercise also directly affect insulin, which is involved in the synthesis of SHBG. So, there are a number of ways by which diet and exercise can reduce the degree of estrogen dominance. This is by far the safer way to go to "balance" your relative estrogen vs. progesterone hormones.

XENOHORMONES AND ENVIRONMENTAL TOXIN REDUCTION:

Our body is built to withstand incredible amounts of stresses and we are able to live even after being exposed to the equivalent of a toxic waste dump over time. For example, although we are moving into a new era with better and more targeted treatments, the way we treat cancer today is by using very powerful drugs called chemotherapy. These drugs make you puke, lose nerve sensation, cause diarrhea and make all your hair fall out because they are poisons! The only reason this strategy works is because cancer cells are damaged and die more readily than normal cells. So, after each dose more cancer dies but your body rebuilds. This is great, but it does not mean that in the absence of a life-threatening disease, where such drastic measures are required to save your life, that you have to poison yourself daily with all sorts of known toxins. Stop abusing the privilege of being built extra solid like a Mack truck to withstand attacks. Stop waging war on your own body and limit toxin exposure as much as possible.

Other than the idea of staying away from toxins for better general health, why is this being mentioned in a book about ovarian cysts? Many of these toxins contain what are known as "xenohormones" or "endocrine disruptors." These substances look like natural hormones and can attach to the same receptors on your cells, causing either a blockage or an increased effect on the cell. Since there are literally thousands of these out there, we do not yet have a handle on which does what or when. You can bet it is not good.

The problem is that technically many of these toxins are approved by the FDA and other government agencies for use, and this is based largely on "acute toxicity." In other words, how much of it do you have to consume or get exposed to before you drop dead right here, right now. Well, from that perspective, you would have to consume pounds or gallons of many of these toxins over a short time period to drop dead on the spot. The amounts contained in any of the items listed below are truly micro-tiny…almost not measurable, and certainly not even remotely close to pounds or gallons. However, these xenohormones are definitely VERY bioactive (i.e. a micro-tiny amount can affect your hormone balance) AND, to make it worse, they bioaccumulate. This means they get stored in your fat cells, are released erratically and can be constantly bombarding your hormone receptors even though you have not touched that particular item (e.g. plastic bottle) for weeks.

Xenohormones include:

- Growth hormones given to livestock and poultry
- Bisphenol A (BPA): found in polycarbonate resins and hard plastics which often line the containers which hold our soft drinks and food
- Phthalates: which are often found in inks, adhesives, vinyl flooring, some paints and plastics
- Alkylphenols & nonylphenols: found in many detergents, cosmetics, pesticides, shampoos, some clear plastics and spermicidal lubricants. Unfortunately, these are not filtered out in municipal water treatment plants very well, so they can re-enter the food chain and you can be exposed to it over and over. Unfortunately, it is often found in tap water in the US.

Here's an intimate tip regarding exposure to several xenohormones that you might not even be thinking about. It turns out that quite a few sex toys contain them. Although a bit dated by now, the Danish Environmental Protection Agency released a report in 2006 which helps distinguish which ones do and how to find out.

There are many others. You can certainly make a list and try to avoid all of this. A good resource is the Environmental Working Group (https://ewg.org), which categorizes many products as to toxin levels and safety.

Unfortunately, it is impossible to avoid all toxins, even if you reside in a rural outpost living off your own land, way off the grid. Nonetheless, you can reduce your exposure. You should know these toxins are out there, they are ubiquitous, they are potent, and they can be messing with your body's hormonal delicate balance. Certainly, you can take a look at the list above and take some general action. For example, stay away from pesticides, non-organic dairy, meat and poultry. You can also use porcelain and heat tempered glass rather than plastic to heat your food. These are but a few tips, but you get the idea. There are ways to at least reduce this threat.

SUPERCHARGING YOUR DETOX-ABILITY

Can you do anything to improve your body's ability to defend itself against toxins, so that you can reduce this risk from xenohormones? After all, your body is already a great detox machine. It was designed that way, and boy is that great in this day of toxins galore! But the answer is clear. You can definitely amplify your detox-ability a *lot*! Your main detox engine is the liver, which we are going to concentrate on. But keep in mind that your kidneys, lungs and skin also help clear your system of toxins.

An occasional or even a rather frequent periodic "detoxification" or "cleanse" has become a very popular, but misunderstood, means of trying to proactively "stay healthy" and "boost energy." Some gurus recommend detox on a "seasonal" basis or some equally arbitrary non-scientific recommendation. This may initially involve a liver detox "kit," a colon cleanse, an elimination diet or many other options. However, did you know that this periodic regimen is robbing you of optimal health and longevity? It's easier than you think to get into a constant energy and health-boosting daily detox lifestyle. No more ups and downs!

So what's the secret? Well, your body's normal detox processes occur at the cellular, molecular and even epigenetic level. Huh? Don't worry, while it's important for you to understand why this is important, it is not necessary for you to become a molecular biologist or doctor or anything like that. However, we do live in a modern world and the scientific level of understanding about how the human body works is now at a very deep level. By reading this, you are setting yourself apart from the crowd.

So, isn't an intermittent detoxification or cleanse enough? No! Your body moves along on a biological time-clock measured by seconds to minutes, not days to months. An occasional detox "tune-up" won't cut it. This is especially true if you live the high paced partly junk food and entertainment "good life" between your detox tune-ups.

Liver Detox Potentiation

Taking some supplements can theoretically help enhance some liver detoxification processes, and provide antioxidant protection from free radicals. The question is how much supplementation in each individual is really needed. It is plausible to consider supplementation based on the nature of the biochemical detox reactions, but the details are simply not worked out with respect to risk vs. benefit. In moderation, this is highly unlikely to cause harm and the theoretical, or proven upside is huge. As a general rule, whenever you can get these nutrients from diet… you should.

Fish Oils And Omega Fatty Acids

The detox effects related to fish oil are based on limiting inflammation, which can lead to increased internal metabolic toxin production and chronic disease. Even though Omega-3 fatty acids are anti-inflammatory and Omega-6 fatty acids are pro-inflammatory, they are both considered "good" and essential for you in the right balance. Fish oils from wild cold water fish are the best-balanced source since wild fish eat more algae which are a rich source of the Omega-3 variant. Recommended total fish oil dose ranges from 1 gram/day to 2-4 grams/day. However, be careful. Excess intake can lead to intestinal disturbances, bleeding, and in very high doses even Omega-3 fatty acids become oxidants. In that case, antioxidants are recommended including vitamins C, E, and selenium, which are sometimes found packaged together in a capsule for this reason. The best strategy is not to overdo it.

If fish oil supplements are your choice over fresh fish, keep in mind that the dosing is NOT all the same despite similar looking labels. A one gram(1g) capsule of fish oil typically contains about 120 mg of docosahexaenoic acid (DHA) and 180 mg of eicosapentaenoic acid (EPA), but the total amount of Omega-3 can vary from 100 to 300mg per gram depending upon the type of fish oil.

The best marine sources of Omega fatty acids are lower on the food chain. Along those lines, New Zealand Green Lipped Mussels or Krill, which is a tiny shrimp-like organism, are some of the best. The higher you go up in the food chain, the more likely it may be contaminated with Mercury and other toxins. Of course, supplements are often monitored for toxins, but if you are looking at dietary intake, this is something to consider. Also, unless you have several million dollars worth of testing equipment in your kitchen, you will never know if the toxin levels are as reported on the supplement bottle or not.

Finally, you can also supplement your Omega-3 needs from flaxseed, which contains about 700mg per gram of oil in the form of alpha-linolenic acid. Other plant sources include green leafy vegetables, algae, soybeans and hemp seeds.

These are not considered to be as good for heart health as marine sources, but they are still a good option overall.

Alpha Lipoic Acid (ALA)

Alpha-lipoic acid is an antioxidant that is made and found in practically every cell in the body, where it also helps turn glucose into energy. This should not be confused with another ALA, which is alpha-linolenic acid, an Omega-3 fatty acid. Unlike other antioxidants, which work only in water (e.g. Vitamin C) or fatty tissues (e.g. Vitamin E), alpha-lipoic acid is both fat – and water-soluble and can work throughout the body. It assists synthesis of glutathione, which is a potent antioxidant and helps the liver with detoxification.

In general, a healthy body makes enough ALA, but supplementation might help fight damaging free radicals and the dose range generally reported is between 100 and 600 mg per day. Animal models have shown ALA to have a protective role against heavy metal or chemical toxicity.

Vitamin C

Ascorbic acid is a storied vitamin. Unfortunately, there are many exaggerations along with the scientifically proven or plausible effects. As far as enhancing detox-ability, vitamin C is an antioxidant and free radical scavenger, which means that it neutralizes them. Like ALA it helps increase glutathione synthesis, which you remember is important as part of Phase II liver detox.

As far as dosage, this is where part of the hype and exaggeration comes in. Grams and grams of vitamin C may lead to more side effects and toxicity than benefit. At approximately 500mg per day, 63% is absorbed. Absorption of powder is most efficient. Your tissues will achieve all that they need at about 200mg/day for a relatively short period, which is individual. Beyond this amount, the excess is simply passed into the urine.

Vitamin D

Regarding detox specifically, vitamin D has recently been discovered to help dial down fat. In that way, it can reduce the amount of toxins bioaccumulating in your body. Vitamin D can also directly affect upper respiratory infections, rheumatoid arthritis, multiple sclerosis, type 2 diabetes, and has an anti-cancer effect.

Vitamin D is synthesized by the skin when exposed to sunlight but is activated in the kidney assuming enough magnesium is present. A solid day in the sun, assuming you did not block it all, can produce 10,000 to 25,000 International Units (IU) of vitamin D. Having said that, please avoid sunburn as this can lead to a skin cancer called melanoma, which is deadly. Also, keep in mind that many people who live in the "sun belt" are still deficient.

Assuming your sun exposure is not consistently at a high level on an every-day basis, supplementation is best. The Institute of Medicine has recently raised the daily minimum requirement recommendation to the range of 600-800IU daily, depending on age and sex. However, other expert organizations feel that is too low based on best evidence. A range of 2000IU to 10,000IU per day leads to the following effects: 1) promotes fat metabolism by reducing parathyroid hormone output and increasing fat breakdown by the liver, 2) activates receptors on fat cells, suppressing fat cell growth, 3) increases sensitivity to leptin, which tells your brain that you are not hungry, and 4) reduces fat accumulation in muscles. If you are not sure that you have "enough" circulating vitamin D, you can have it measured. Levels of 30-50ng/ml are considered sufficient to optimal, but it can be reported in different units. So beware of that when comparing results. The best strategy is to get your blood tested and not exceed the normal range. Liver toxicity can occur at really high levels.

Vitamin E

Otherwise known as alpha-tocopherol, vitamin E is a fat-soluble vitamin and is a potent antioxidant, which is critical to daily detox activity and may support liver cell health. The average dose is 400IU per day and is best absorbed with meals. Excess dosage can thin your blood and make you prone to bruising and bleeding. This is why the upper limit recommended dose is between 1000 and 1500 IU. While this might be one of the least toxic of the fat soluble vitamins, other side effects like intestinal disturbances, weakness, fatigue and double vision have been reported. Also, there is no data that says more is better.

Magnesium

Magnesium is an earth metal element essential to the human diet. Over 300 enzymes require magnesium to function properly, including those in the liver. It is also critical for the formation of cyclic adenosine monophosphate (cAMP) which helps move ions across cell membranes. Rich sources include spices, nuts, cereals, coffee, cocoa, tea, and vegetables including green leafy vegetables such as spinach. Aging, excessive chronic alcohol intake and stress increase requirements. Magnesium citrate is available as the most bio-available oral supplement, but the dose varies. Higher doses (3-5 grams) can cause diarrhea and resulting dehydration. Ideally, replacement should be done based on lab values showing you are deficient. Although it is not a toxin, very aggressive dosing can cause you to stop breathing because at high concentrations it paralyzes muscle. It's a better strategy to maintain levels based on adequate intake of the foods mentioned above. Due to kidney regulation, it is almost impossible to overdose on dietary amounts, but it is certainly possible with aggressive supplementation.

Selenium

Selenium is an essential trace element. It represents a great example of how a toxic chemical is essential to life, and it is all a matter of degree. In tiny quantities, it is essential for cellular function and specifically for glutathione peroxidase enzyme activity in Phase II detox. In larger quantities, it is toxic and increases cellular oxidation. Good dietary sources include garlic, broccoli, onions and Brazil nuts. The daily dose range is 100 to 200 micro-grams, which can be accomplished by consuming one or two Brazil nuts. At only 910 micrograms acute toxicity symptoms like nausea and vomiting can occur, and a few grams (still a pretty small amount) is deadly.

Glutathione

Glutathione is a vital antioxidant tri-peptide (i.e. essentially a tiny protein) and helps protect cells against free radicals and peroxides. In fact, the ratio of reduced glutathione to oxidized glutathione within cells is often used as a measure of cellular toxicity status. It is synthesized within the body. Glutathione is crucial for liver detox function.

The best source of supplemental glutathione is through consuming fruits and vegetables. Taking synthetic supplement formulations is not recommended as they are not very bioavailable. Intestinal and liver enzymes deactivate them readily.

Taurine

Also known as 2-aminoethanesulfonic acid, taurine is an amino acid which is synthesized in the pancreas and then conjugated to become a component of bile. From a detox perspective, it stimulates bile flow. It is also an antioxidant and scavenges free radicals. It tends to be present in lower concentrations in vegans. So, even though it is not essential in the diet, if one were looking to optimize their detox plan it can be supplemented. Average dose reported in studies is 2 grams per day, taken in three divided doses.

SAMe

S-adenosyl methionine is a chemical compound synthesized and used throughout the body, but mostly in the liver. It is a "methyl group donor" in the chemical process of detox by methylation (e.g. one of Phase II reaction types in the liver). It is also helpful in bile flow stimulation and can help regenerate glutathione when levels fall. Nutrients required for its synthesis are choline, folic acid, and vitamin B12. Concentrations decrease with age.

Supplementation dose range for liver disease is 400-1600 mg per day, best absorbed on an empty stomach. However, be very careful if you have bipolar disorder or Parkinson's disease. Also, there are possible other severe side effects if vitamin B6, vitamin B12, and folic acid levels are inadequate. These include increased risk of heart attacks, strokes, liver damage, and possibly Alzheimer's disease.

SAMe supplementation can also produce anxiety, insomnia, various intestinal side effects and dry mouth. This can occur with as little as 50mg per day supplementation. Based on this, perhaps the better strategy for many people is to maintain cofactor B vitamin supplementation and depend on your own body's synthesis of SAMe. Otherwise, it is best to consider this supplementation only under medical supervision.

Milk Thistle

Otherwise known as Sylibum marianum, milk thistle is a flowering plant native to the Mediterranean region. It has been used for over 2000 years to help various liver problems. With modern science, we know that the active component is silymarin, which contains four flavonolignans. These are powerful antioxidants and enhance liver regeneration. The dose range is 140-210 mg per day of Milk Thistle, assuming it contains 70-80% silymarin.

Schisandra

Otherwise known as Schisandra chinensis, the fruit of schisandra contains the active flavonolignans which have the anti-inflammatory and anti-oxidant effects.

Schisandra also improves liver detox by improving Phase II enzyme activity. The dose range is 500-1500mg per day of boiled schisandra tea.

Dandelion

Taraxum officinale may improve digestion and stimulates bile flow, while also exhibiting antioxidant and anti-inflammatory activity. Its leaves also contain various vitamins and minerals, especially vitamins A, C and K, calcium and potassium, among others. The entire plant has beneficial effects, and the dose ranges are as follows: leaf 4-10mg tea three times per day, root 2-8mg tea three times per day. As with any form of herbal or prescription substance, there may be adverse side effects. For example, at low doses, it may help prevent cancer, but at higher doses, it can promote cancer. Any bile flow stimulants should be consumed with caution in people who have gallbladder or bile duct conditions.

Artichoke

Cynara cardunculus has also been shown to contain compounds that are bile flow stimulants. These include chlorogenic acid, scolymoside, caffeoylquinic acid and cynarine. The dose range of leaf extract preparations is about 600mg three times per day. Or, just eat artichokes which is easier.

Water Fasting

To avoid confusion, please keep in mind that "intermittent fasting" which is very short and down to a twelve-hour eating window, or caloric restriction are not the same as fasting for days or a week or more. Intermittent fasting and caloric restriction do have some health benefits. Prolonged fasting reduces the liver's ability to detoxify because nutritional depletion lowers production of enzymes. So, do not fast for detoxification and "cleansing" purposes. You will lose far more than you will gain.

Fasting is often recommended as part of an intermittent detox regimen and is defined as a period with water intake only. Keep in mind that if juices are involved, this is a modified fast and may lead to very different results. Also, bear in mind that toxins are more absorbable on an empty stomach, so keep additional chemical exposure to a minimum.

While there is a scientific theoretical basis for brief fasting, it comes with some drawbacks. First of all, when you fast your body rapidly runs out of glucose from your muscle glycogen stores. Other than possibly feeling run down until your body converts to burning your fat stores, your brain screams out and you are likely to experience headaches. When you convert to fat burning for energy you become ketogenic, and the brain has to learn how to run on ketones and not glucose, its preferred fuel. This can take a few days before your brain gets used to it, and this results in headache *pain*! Who needs it? It can be avoided if you approach detox as a daily habit rather than a periodic and unnecessary shocking stress on your body.

So what is the theoretical basis for fasting during periodic detox? Toxins bioaccumulate in your fat cells. Upon starting a detox regimen, these toxins can be released into the bloodstream at a more rapid rate as you burn the fat they are hiding in. So a temporary additional increase in symptoms (i.e. beyond those caused by ketones) can occur because more toxins may be circulating in your body. These symptoms can include fatigue or malaise and just feeling ill. First recognized in the treatment of syphilis, it is known as the Jarisch-Herxheimer reaction and may also occur during parasitic and fungal infections. As the infecting organisms die, their internal and external parts (exo and endotoxins) cause a severe inflammatory reaction with fevers and muscle pain, much like you would experience with the flu. This type of reaction has not been proven with removal of accumulated chemical xenobiotic toxins in your fat cells but remains a theoretical consideration. The reason I mention this is that damage that occurs at the cellular level may be quite severe but not recognized by your body enough to produce acute symptoms. So, even though you may not feel it, bad things can be happening at the cellular level.

So, as in everything else, moderation in approaching detoxification is reasonable. Since we are talking about a long-term detoxification process here for maximum safe effect, there is no reason to risk bad effects by jumping in too fast and too aggressively. First of all, the total toxin amount that you might theoretically purge from fat cells by periodic detox is relatively small unless you intend to mobilize all of your fat in 3-4 days. Of course, this is impossible. Also, instead of periodically risking side effects and increased damage to your cells (which then need repair) why not reduce the amount of fat you carry by longer term strategies of diet and exercise? Although this violates the popular fitness concept of " no pain, no gain," the reality is that in almost all systems continued maintenance is better than periodic emergency shock therapy. As an example, this is true in a simple system like maintaining chlorine levels in your swimming pool. Shocking a pool with high concentrations of chlorine destroys the walls of the pool over time and makes it unusable for periods of time. It is much better to keep the chlorine level in balance. If it's true in this simple pool example, it is certainly true for an infinitely more complex system like your body.

Microbiome and Probiotics

Probiotics are part of the discussion related to many aspects of optimizing health, including detox. Your "microbiome", which is represented by all the bacteria living on your skin and inside of you, contain at least 3X more bacterial cells than your own cells. So, there is far more of "them" than "you" in you. For those that are germaphobes that may come as a shock but these bacteria help you in many ways including fighting off bad bacteria and helping metabolize toxins. More importantly, related to the topic of this book, part of your intestinal microbiome is called the estrobolome. This helps balance your estrogen. When you have more "bad gut bugs" growing, possibly due to an unhealthy diet or having taken antibiotics, they produce an enzyme called betaglucuronidase. This enzyme essentially contributes to recycling of estrogen rather than healthy excretion, increasing your estrogen levels. This is another way that estrogen dominance can occur.

Rather than lathering on more bio-identical progesterone to balance the estrogen dominance, in addition to the other techniques we've already covered, keeping your gut microbiome healthy will lead to a healthy estrobolome, help detoxify you and reduce excess estrogen. This is based on science that is literally hot off the presses over the last few years. So, either consume a healthy dose of fermented foods (eg. Kombucha) or take probiotics and the prebiotics that feed them. Not long into the future, based on developing studies, we will be able to test individuals and recommend specific probiotics. That day is not here yet, although some labs are dabbling in offering something that is not yet ready for prime time. Also, there is no evidence that more is better in terms of the number of colony forming units (CFU) supplement manufacturers use. Seven core genera of probiotics often included in products are Lactobacillus, Bifidobacterium, Saccharomyces, Streptococcus, Enterococcus, Escherichia, and Bacillus. For now, either consume probiotics in your diet or buy a name-brand mix of probiotics, prebiotics, and synbiotics from your health food and supplement store.

Summary Daily Detoxification Plan

In summary, effective detoxification is based on daily maintenance that will contribute to steady high energy levels and improved health. Limiting your external toxin exposure as much as possible and improving your body's detox-ability will reduce xenohormone influence and likely add years if not decades of healthy vibrant life.

On a *daily* basis your new three step detox solution habits are:

Avoid external toxins

- Shop for non-toxin laden organic foods and personal care items
- Research before you buy & use household cleaning and maintenance items
- Monitor your environment and avoid those things that seem "unnatural" as much as possible. If you can't read what is on the label (i.e. long chemical names) it's probably not good for you.

Reduce internal toxin production

- Low glycemic index, anti-inflammatory, antioxidant rich diet
- Exercise daily 20-30 minutes cardio minimum

Improve your detox-ability through

- Daily bowel movements
- Diaphragmatic deep breathing exercises daily
- Hydration
- Selected nutrients, supplements and herbals
- Probiotics & Prebiotics

Your body will appreciate you for your continued daily attention rather than periodic shock therapy like a pool might get with a chlorine shock pack. A daily detox routine is what is most likely to get you to a long healthy life, and may help keep ovarian cysts away as a bonus.

Natural Symptom Control

Compresses and Aromatherapy

Warm compresses decrease muscle cramping in an injured area, and it generally feels good. However, lest you think you are warming up your ovaries, they are at least 8 inches deep. It is not likely that you can get heat that deep from a hot compress, even if it were boiling hot. Obviously, this would not be recommended since you would burn your skin. Still, warm compresses can be very soothing and de-stressing if you are in pain or discomfort.

Essential oils that have been recommended to apply to the skin near the pelvis include rosemary, lavender and chamomile. Combining these with massage will reduce some of the muscle tension that adds to pelvic and ovarian pain. Although not proven, it is felt that some essential oils may actually activate your brain's endorphins, which act as natural painkillers. More on this in the next section.

Cold DECREASES circulation and causes muscle spasm. That is why you get frostbite and you hear about people's fingers and toes falling off. This is not a good idea other than a way to rapidly reduce swelling in sports injuries. Stick with warm for pelvic pain.

Exercise

In order to optimize your body's hormonal balance, especially if you need to knock off more than a few pounds, a structured exercise program is one of the best things you can do. I know what you're thinking, "I'm in pain, I can't go bouncing around and giving myself more pain!" That may be true, but here is a good reason to do it anyway and a few tips as to how.

When you exercise, you produce biochemicals in your brain called endorphins.

This is your body's "natural morphine" which can bring you pain relief and a natural high of sorts. After about 10 minutes of moderate exercise you are on the way. About the bouncing around problem: try low impact exercise like walking, swimming or even yoga.

Here's a tip that may be worth the price of this whole book. Instead of having to take powerful painkilling narcotics, you can extend the activity of your endorphins by taking DLPA or DL-Phenylalanine. This is a natural essential amino acid that you can buy over the counter at your friendly health food and supplements store. DLPA has been in the medical spotlight for chronic pain and depression. It has also helped with symptoms of PMS. How? It slows down enzymes that "eat up" endorphins so that the level you built up with your 10 minutes or more of exercise stays up longer, providing extended pain relief. This is not like taking a pain pill, because it does not work in minutes. It generally takes almost a month to notice a difference, so it is a long-term play. Also, by itself, DLPA won't do anything. So, no excuses. Get up off that couch. You'll be glad you did. Oh, and as always, talk with your doctor before taking DLPA. If you are pregnant or have certain conditions, like phenylketonuria [PKU], you should not take DLPA.

In addition, yoga and tai chi specifically focus on stress reduction, muscle relaxation, improved circulation and awareness building for a form of pain reducing biofeedback. You simply can't go wrong here.

If you exercise outside, you pick up some Vitamin D from the sun's healing rays. Vitamin D is critical to many body balancing processes, including those related to hormones. But be careful…don't get a sunburn. Better to take a supplement or dairy products if you are ok with them. The problem with many dairy products is that they may contain estrogens and xenoestrogens. The proper dose of Vitamin D depends on blood levels that can easily be measured. But you can't go wrong with at least 1000IU per day. Best to measure.

Acupuncture and Acupressure

This Chinese eons-old practice involves inserting long, extremely fine thin needles into specific points in the skin. In the modern version, this can be combined with electrical stimulation (electro-acupuncture) for even better results. Stimulation with pinpoint pressure massage, acupressure, can also achieve pain relief by targeting trigger points. Combining this technique with Western medicine, these trigger points can also be injected with pain medications.

Massage

While a general massage might help relieve stress and feels good, a specific kind can take off where standard acupressure leaves off. A form of Japanese massage called Shiatsu actually means "finger pressure". Although there are a number of variations of this massage technique it generally addresses entire meridians (energy channels) in your body rather than specific trigger points. True master practitioners are beyond basic massage therapist level, so you need to seek out those who practice this specific art well. When you find a master, there are stretching routines they can teach you to do yourself.

There are no Western controlled studies that prove this works or that "qi" basis for it exists, but case reports and anecdotal evidence suggest something is working to relieve pain.

If you want to try something yourself, there are two points which generally affect the pelvic area, mostly related to menstrual pain and PMS. You can use your index finger and middle finger to exert moderate force and pressure on these points. The first is called the Sea of Energy and is located two finger-breadths below your belly button. The second is on the outside of your leg, three finger breadths below the knee cap. Try this one sitting down. Remember, it took master practitioners years to get it right, so don't get discouraged if it doesn't work right away. Get some help.

Biofeedback

You can control pain by responding to gentle visual and sound stimulation cues which cause you to relax and de-stress. You specifically learn to relax specific muscles which may be tense and causing pain. Practitioners even use special vaginal tampons which measure the response so that you can see your progress. When it works, it seems to work very well according to case reports and testimonials.

Hypnotism

You have certainly heard of this technique no doubt, but probably did not think it would help. Those that are susceptible to hypnosis and can achieve the altered state of consciousness can learn how to distract themselves using psychologically implanted cues. Self hypnosis takes a while to master but has been reported to work even if you are only moderately "suggestible".

Psycho-Neuro-Immunology

We know that stress influences a lot of body functions and normal reproductive cycling is one of them. This is not just a loose psychological association but rather there are very specific scientific explanations for this, involving hormone balance.

Psychological stress physically kicks off a hormone cascade leading to all of the metabolic abnormalities already discussed which lead to PCOS and, to some extent, physiologic cyst formation in general. How does it do that? The origins are in our subconscious "fight or flight" response. When confronted with the stress of a threat our body quickly starts secreting stress hormones which increase heart rate, blood pressure and muscle tension. We are then physically ready to fight or run away, depending upon what the best option is at the time. Although this is a great short-term response, if you are under chronic stress, elevation of the same stress hormones (e.g. cortisol, adrenaline) are not good for you in any way.

Further research into the "fight or flight" response led to the birth of "psychoneuroimmunology" (PNI) as a science. Of course, mind-body techniques have been around for eons, but we are looking at bridging East-West these days for a more holistic solution. So, this means there is now a mainstream research medicine approach that looks at the connection between thoughts, emotions, the brain, the nervous system and your immune system. This means you can basically think and feel your way into disease, or at least contribute to it. The good news is that it goes both ways. You can also use mind-body techniques to think and feel your way OUT of disease, or at least help yourself heal.

The main goal is to de-stress. There are tons of techniques out there that include mind and/or body exercises. Learned relaxation response can be achieved by yoga, Quigong, meditation, aromatherapy, music, massage and many others. The main effect you would ideally like to achieve is a carryover beyond the relaxation session. In other words, the techniques you learn in sessions should help you stay calm throughout the day. That is the ultimate goal. In the evening, a good night's sleep is medically therapeutic. It is not just a matter to feeling "fresh." It is a matter of biochemistry and the imbalancing effect on hormones if you are not asleep during the best part of your sleep-wake cycle, which is between 10PM and 3AM. Six to eight hours of sleep, including this time period, is best. If you can't sleep well, before resorting to drugs, try Melatonin, which is a natural supplement that helps many. Start with a very low dose and work upwards.

Stress response is also reduced by a number of herbals, including extracts of kava, valerian, Phellodendron and Magnolia, which reduce anxiety and insomnia. On the other hand, caffeine interferes with sleep and is a stressor. So coffee, tea and caffeinated sodas are something to stay away from. Clearly stay away from stress inducing toxins like smoking.

Systems of care: Similarities and Differences

If you read between the lines, there are some common threads between the various alternative viewpoints, and some even align with Western mainstream medical thought.

- Traditional Chinese medicine (TCM) uses acupuncture, acupressure, dietary and herbal remedies for ovarian cysts.
- Ayurvedic medicine focuses on herbal remedies, diet, exercise, yoga, massage, and detoxification. (**NOTE**: We could not find anything worth writing about in terms of "detoxification" cleanses to treat ovarian cysts. Keep the toxins out by paying attention to what you drink and eat or put on your body, including skincare creams and shampoos. Otherwise your body is GREAT at detoxifying itself and anything you add could harm you by washing important vitamins, minerals and body fluids out in the process….not to mention possible mechanical injury and toxicity from the stuff that is in these quasi-miraculous cleanses. We don't recommend this approach for treating ovarian cysts at this time. Detox is an ongoing lifestyle choice, not a quick fix cleanse.)
- Homeopathic medicine suggests "like treats like", or the law of similars. Specific recommendations are Apis Mellifica [The Honey-bee, Bee sting] for right ovarian cysts…ouch…. and Colocynthis [Bitter Cucumber, Colocy, Colocynth] for left ovarian cysts, and general hormone and

immune system balancing. (**NOTE**: Herbal remedies and homoeopathic remedies are not the same thing. The idea behind homeopathy is determining what substance, in an infinitesimally tiny amount, would produce the same symptoms that you might be experiencing. That substance, in the very tiny amount, is exactly what you take. These remedies are usually based on herbs, or other ingredients. However homeopathic remedies are diluted until there is only a tiny trace amount of the original herbal ingredients left. These remedies are also not prescribed like mainstream drugs, which are given to "counter" the disease or symptoms. A common example of homeopathy for pain, including postoperative pain, is Arnica gel applied to the skin. In normal doses it is a very toxic herb. But in highly diluted homeopathic gels it helps some patients. Is the data strong? No. But there is no downside to external application in dilute doses. Do not take it internally as it can be toxic at any dose.

- Naturopathy aligns somewhat with Western medicine and views ovarian cysts as being related to insulin resistance and blood sugar problems. They advocate dietary remedies, herbs and supplements to balance hormones and insulin levels.

Premenstrual Syndrome

Some of the symptoms you may be having and attributing to ovarian cysts may actually be related to PMS, which is a very real hormone-based problem. Here are some tips for coping with premenstrual syndrome.

- Calcium: 1,200 to 1,500 milligrams (mg) of dietary and supplemental calcium per day helps reduce both physical and psychological symptoms. It's also good for your bones.
- Magnesium: 400 mg per day in supplement form can help decrease fluid retention, bloating and breast tenderness
- Vitamin B-6: 50 to 100 mg per day, especially if you are on birth control pills.
- Vitamin E: 400 international units (IU) per day, can reduce prostaglandin production. These act like hormones which cause breast tenderness and cramps.
- Herbal supplements: Various herbs have been reported to help, but there is very little scientific evidence that any one is better than the other, but there is very little downside to trying. These include: CBD oil, black cohosh, ginger, raspberry leaf, dandelion, chasteberry and evening primrose oil.
- Bio-Identical or Natural progesterone: Most often the recommendation is for cream, but it is also available in pill form. Bio-Identical progesterone is derived from wild yams and soybeans. Some women swear by them, but there is no good scientific evidence that this works. Also, keep in mind that compounding pharmacies are not well regulated, so the dose you take may not be what is on the label. Consider the balancing strategies discussed earlier in this book to reduce estrogen instead.

**Important: Please check with your health care provider before consuming any herbs or dietary supplements.

Minimally Invasive Ovarian Surgery

If surgery is determined to be the best option, mainly because it is probably an ovarian cystic tumor and not a physiologic ovarian cyst, then the goal is to safely perform the surgery and to help you recover as quickly as possible. Emergency surgery can also be done minimally invasively, in case of torsion or cyst rupture with bleeding. The old school way of performing surgery is through a rather large skin incision, which may be up and down (vertical), of variable length, or across (transverse, bikini-cut or C-section) the lower abdomen. Both significantly disturb and traumatize the abdominal wall, not to mention lead to large scars. Vertical incisions are prone to falling apart, getting infected and to form hernias down the line. Bikini cut transverse incisions heal better and are less prone to hernias but may not be appropriate for a larger cyst that extends upwards into the upper pelvic area or up to the belly button or beyond. For larger ovarian masses, the surgeon just can't reach up high enough to get the job done safely and effectively. In both cases, the pain afterwards is significant and usually it means you stay in the hospital for at least a day or two, and usually more.

Minimally invasive surgery, otherwise known as keyhole or band-aid or belly-button surgery, is performed though much smaller incisions that are as small as the width of a pencil (5 to 8 mm). The number of incisions varies but it can literally be a few or up to five or six, depending upon what it takes to get the job done safely. Some, or sometimes all, can be hidden in the belly button and bikini line. Regardless of how many tiny incisions, this means less trauma, less risk of infection, less risk of hernia, less pain, less blood loss, and so on. The bottom line is that it translates into rapid recovery so that you can go on with life as soon as possible. Most of the time you can go home the same day or the next morning.

There are two main types of minimally invasive ovarian surgery techniques, laparoscopy and robotically assisted laparoscopy. Both are used, both can be effective, but depending on the situation there are key differences. What are these differences and why does it matter?

LAPAROSCOPY

The first laparoscopic surgery on humans was performed in 1910 by a Swedish surgeon, Hans Christian Jacobaeus. So, this technique has been around for over a hundred years and has been refined in many ways. It was not until the 1980's that the cameras, optics and instruments became good enough to routinely perform larger gynecologic surgery, including surgery on the ovaries. It also took a while before the benefits of faster recovery were proven. There is also a learning curve for surgeons, so wide adoption has really occurred mainly over the past few decades or so. Now, more and more surgeons are offering this technique instead of large incision laparotomy surgeries.

While laparoscopy is superior to laparotomy in many ways, it has limitations. First of all the optics are two-dimensional. The surgeon operates by looking at a TV screen and has no real depth perception. This is kind of like driving with one eye closed. It's hard to see what is closer and what is further away. The more complicated the surgery, the more this can lead to errors and surgical injuries.

The second limitation is that the instruments that are introduced through the keyhole incision ports are rigid and straight. The graspers and scissors can only move up and down and side to side. This gets clunky and is reminiscent of operating with chop-sticks. Attempted finesse moves turn into Epic fails because of the limited push-pull, rip-and-tear motions possible. Also, any tremor that the surgeon may have is amplified at the tip of the instruments where the surgery is happening. This goes for the surgeon and the assistant, resulting in some potentially herky-jerky spastic moves. This can lead to unfortunate bleeding and more trauma to delicate tissues. Worse, the fulcrum of the surgery, the pivot point, is at the abdominal wall. This means that the instruments are moved a lot at the incision point in the abdominal wall and can lead to a lot of bruising and tearing of the muscles underneath. This in turn means more postoperative pain, even though it is less than that of a big incision laparotomy.

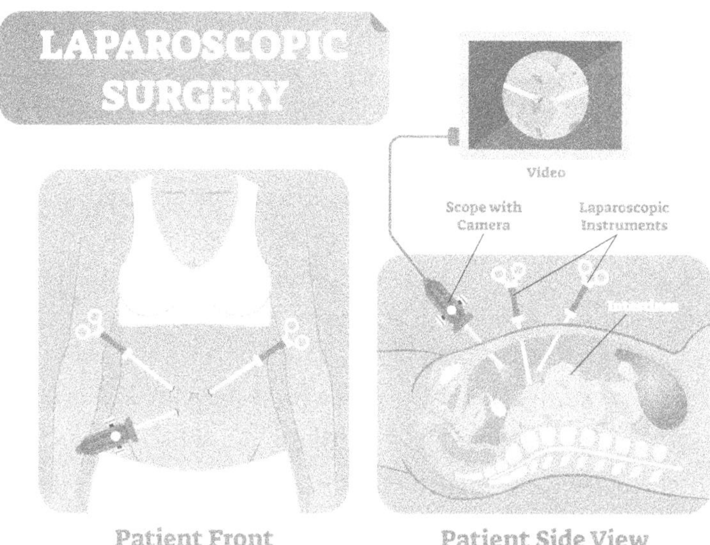

Overall, it is possible to do quite a bit laparoscopically and, especially if the surgery is not too complicated, it is "ok" and good enough. The problem is it is hard to anticipate what will be easy and what will not be easy. So, "just OK…is not OK", because you never know what will be found and your surgeon could be stuck with inadequate resources during surgery. If this happens, the surgery is "converted" to a big incision laparotomy to finish the job.

ROBOTICALLY-ASSISTED LAPAROSCOPY

Robotically assisted surgery takes laparoscopy to the next level in multiple crucial ways. First of all the camera allows the surgeon to see everything in 3D, so the vision is crystal clear with full depth perception.

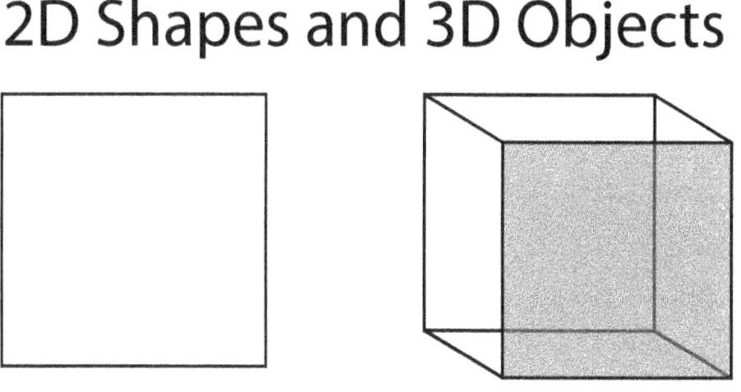

The surgeon knows with exact precision where they are relative to important and delicate structures, down to the millimeter. Secondly the instruments at the tip, where the surgery actually happens, are "wristed", simulating a human hand. The instruments are controlled via a stabilizing system so there is no tremor at the tip of the instruments. This allows for extremely delicate and precise movements, minimizing trauma and injuries. Lastly, the surgeon is in control of three instruments at the same time, allowing the surgeon to assist themselves with stable and non-spastic holding of tissues vs that which happens with a herky-jerky laparoscopic assistant. The bedside surgical assistant still helps under certain circumstances with another grasper or is ready to suction and irrigate if any troublesome bleeding occurs. All of this also results in less motion trauma at the abdominal wall (since the surgery is being done at the instruments tips, not at the abdominal wall fulcrum) and thus the postoperative pain in minimized.

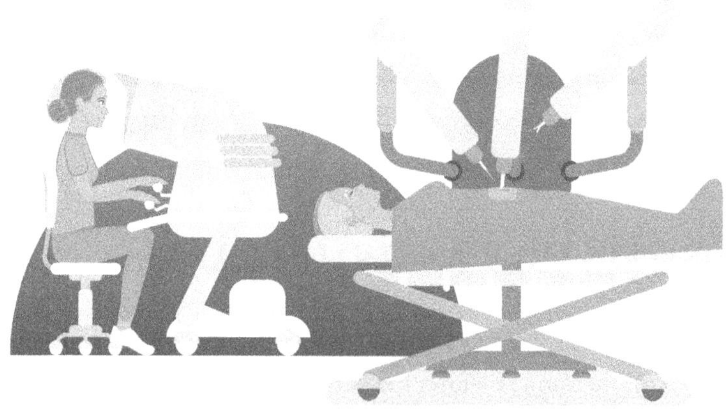

The downside to robotic surgery is that it takes a little longer (minutes), which translates into higher costs for the hospital. But this does not translate to any increased charges for you, so it is simply not a concern for you as the patient. The doctor and hospital are not paid more and the insurance does not charge you more or increase your co-pay. The other minor concern is that the incisions are 8mm vs that of 5mm using most laparoscopic instruments. The 3mm difference is not something you would notice. That is basically a pencil tip. The number of ports can be equivalent to laparoscopy or one or two more. But again, given that they are very small incisions, it generally goes unnoticed by most patients. Safety first.

You may be wondering how a mass can be removed through a keyhole 5 to 8mm incision. The answer is that it usually can't. Depending upon how much of the cyst is fluid vs. solid parts, one of the incisions (usually at the bikini line or hidden in the belly button) is made a little bit larger. Most of the time the cyst or mass is placed in a protective bag, introduced through one of the small ports, and then the mass is removed in the bag. What this does is protect you from spilled contents, whether it be blood in the cyst, hair and thick inflammatory fluid or cancer cells. All of it is trapped in the bag as it is being extracted. There is one exception to making an incision larger for extraction of the cyst, and that is if a hysterectomy is being performed. In these cases, both the uterus and the bag with the cyst or ovarian mass is extracted through the vagina. In fact, when trying to minimize scars in younger and more athletic body-conscious patients, an incision can be made in the vagina behind the uterus to extract the bag. The vaginal incision is closed with sutures and the uterus is left alone. The tradeoff is no larger incisions in the abdomen vs a little longer delay before resuming sexual relations through vaginal intercourse. That is because the stitched area has to heal.

This type of surgery is not just for small ovarian cysts and tumors. Even advanced ovarian cancer surgery can be done in a minimally invasive manner. All of the necessary biopsies can be done using the ports described above. So, "early" ovarian cancer surgery can be and is performed using minimally invasive surgery by many gynecologic oncologists. Advanced ovarian cancer surgery (called cytoreduction or debulking) can be and is performed across the country by a more limited number of gynecologic oncologists who are more expert surgeons, usually using robotically assisted surgery. Optimal or complete cytoreduction is possible (meaning all visible disease is removed) in most patients using advanced techniques and the recovery is vastly superior to a huge midline big vertical incision that usually extends from the chest to the pubic bone. Even when this is not possible using robotics alone, a smaller incision (around 6cm) can be made to allow a human hand to be introduced using a special "hand-port", allowing more flexibility in certain cases. The recovery is still markedly faster than when a full laparotomy larger incision, that can be 20 inches long, is required. More rapid recovery after advanced cancer surgery is not just desirable because you feel better sooner. It is also critical to resume cancer chemo-biotherapy as soon as possible to give you the best chance for a cure. The difference between restarting chemo after minimally invasive vs laparotomy approach can be many weeks if not a month or more.

Yours truly has been successfully performing minimally invasive surgery for over

30 years, including advanced robotics for advanced ovarian cancer and advanced endometriosis for the better part of a decade. Whenever cancer is suspected, or you have had multiple prior surgeries or have advanced endometriosis with probable heavy scarring, I highly recommend finding a robotically capable gynecologic oncologist to help you. As with anything else, be careful. Some have far more experience than others and being "robotically trained" is not the same as being "robotically expert". Ask questions to make sure you feel comfortable with the expertise level.

ENHANCED RECOVERY STRATEGIES

Recovery after minimally invasive surgery is very fast, even for advanced complicated cases. It can be made even faster by using enhanced recovery protocols and strategies. These include nutritional preparation, prevention of blood clots, reduction of pain using techniques that avoid the need for narcotics, and much more. New school surgery is rapidly approaching Star Trek level in many ways, so don't get stuck with an old school "just OK" surgeon. That's just not OK these days because there are too many options if you look around, even if you have insurance restrictions or are having trouble with access. Even many county government-run hospitals now have advanced equipment and great surgeons. Seek out the best you can in your area that will treat you in a holistic manner, offering surgery when needed and observation when surgery is not really required.

References

Abduljabbar HS, Bukhari YA, Al Hachim EG, et al. Review of 244 cases of ovarian cysts. Saudi Med J 2015; 36:834.

Adlercreutz H, Gorbach SL, Goldin BR, Woods MN, Dwyer JT, Hämäläinen E. Estrogen metabolism and excretion in Oriental and Caucasian women.J Natl Cancer Inst. 1994 Jul 20;86(14):1076-82.

Berrino F, Bellati C, Secreto G, Camerini E, Pala V, Panico S, Allegro G, Kaaks R. Reducing bioavailable sex hormones through a comprehensive change in diet: the diet and androgens (DIANA) randomized trial. Cancer Epidemiol Biomarkers Prev. 2001 Jan;10(1):25-33.

Bider D, Maschiach S, Dulitzky M, et al: Clinical, surgical and pathologic findings of adnexal torsion in pregnant and nonpregnant women. Surg Gynecol Obstet 1991; 173:363.

Bottomley C, Bourne T. Diagnosis and management of ovarian cyst accidents. Best Pract Res Clin Obstet Gynaecol 2009; 23:711.

Carruba G, Granata OM, Pala V, Campisi I, Agostara B, Cusimano R, Ravazzolo B, Traina A. A traditional Mediterranean diet decreases endogenous estrogens in healthy postmenopausal women. Nutr Cancer. 2006;56(2):253-9.

Caspi B, Appleman Z, Rabinerson D, et al: The growth pattern of ovarian dermoid cysts: A prospective study in premenopausal and postmenopausal women. Fertil Steril 1997; 68:501.

Caspi B, Lerner-Geva L, Dahan M, et al: A possible genetic factor in the pathogenesis of ovarian dermoid cysts. Gynecol Obstet Invest 2003; 56:2003-2006.

Chen D, Chen SR, Shi XL, Guo FL, Zhu YK, Li S, Cai MX, Deng LH, Xu H. Clinical study on needle-pricking therapy for treatment of polycystic ovarial syndrome The First Affiliated Hospital of Jinan University, Guangzhou 510630, China. Zhongguo Zhen Jiu. 2007 Feb;27(2):99-102.

Comerci Jr JT, Licciardi F, Bergh PA, et al: Mature cystic teratoma: A clinico-pathologic evaluation of 517 cases and review of the literature. Obstet Gynecol 1994; 84:22.

Danish EPA: Survey of chemical substances in consumer products no. 77, 2006

Dische FE, Ritche JM: Luteoma of pregnancy. J Pathol 1970; 100:77.

Dottino PR, Levine DA, Ripley DL, Cohen CJ: Laparoscopic management of adnexal masses in premenopausal and postmenopausal women. Obstet Gynecol 1999; 93:223.

Ekerhovd E, Wienerroith H, Staudach A, et al: Preoperative assessment of unilocular adnexal cysts by transvaginal ultrasonography: A comparison between ultrasonographic morphologic imaging and histopatholigic diagnosis. Am J Obstet Gynecol 2001; 184:48.

Farshchi H, Rane A, Love A, Kennedy RL. Diet and nutrition in polycystic ovary syndrome (PCOS): pointers for nutritional management. J Obstet Gynaecol. 2007 Nov;27(8):762-73.

Givens V, Mitchell GE, Harraway-Smith C, et al. Diagnosis and management of adnexal masses. Am Fam Physician 2009; 80:815.

Goldin BR, Adlercreutz H, Dwyer JT, Swenson L, Warram JH, Gorbach SL Effect of diet on excretion of estrogens in pre- and postmenopausal women. Cancer Res. 1981 Sep;41(9 Pt 2):3771-3.

Grimes DA, Jones LB, Lopez LM, Schulz KF. Oral contraceptives for functional ovarian cysts. Cochrane Database Syst Rev. Oct 18 2006;(4):CD006134.

Hahn S, Haselhorst U, Tan S, Quadbeck B, Schmidt M, Roesler S, Kimmig R, Mann K, Janssen OE. Low serum 25-hydroxyvitamin D concentrations are associated with insulin resistance and obesity in women with polycystic ovary syndrome. Exp Clin Endocrinol Diabetes. 2006 Nov;114(10):577-83.

Hallatt JG, Steele CH, Snyder M: Ruptured corpus luteum with hemoperitoneum: A study of 173 surgical cases. Am J Obstet Gynecol 1984; 149:5.

Hartge P, Hayes R, Reding D, et al: Complex ovarian cysts in postmenopausal women are not associated with ovarian cancer risk factors. Am J Obstet Gynecol 2000; 183:1232.

Havrilesky LJ, Peterson BL, Dryden DK, et al: Predictors of clinical outcomes in the laparoscopic management of adnexal masses. Obstet Gynecol 2003; 102:243.

Hou LH, Yang XM, Erkkola R, Wu XK. Therapeutic effects of Jinqi Jiangtang tablet on women with polycystic ovary syndrome. Department of Obstetrics and Gynecology, The First Affiliated Hospital, Heilongjiang University of Chinese Medicine, Harbin, Heilongjiang Province 150040, China. Zhong Xi Yi Jie He Xue Bao. 2006 Nov;4(6):579-84.

Judd HL, Shamonki IM, Frumar AM, Lagasse LD Origin of serum estradiol in postmenopausal women. Obstet Gynecol. 1982 Jun;59(6):680-6.

Kalman DS, Feldman S, Feldman R, Schwartz HI, Krieger DR, Garrison R. Effect of a proprietary Magnolia and Phellodendron extract on stress levels in healthy women: a pilot, double-blind, placebo-controlled clinical trial. Nutr J. 2008 Apr 21;7:11.

Knudsen UB, Tabor A, Mosgaard B, et al: Management of ovarian cysts. Acta Obstet Gynecol Scand 2004; 83:1012.

Koshiba H. Severe chemical peritonitis caused by spontaneous rupture of an ovarian mature cystic teratoma: a case report. J Reprod Med 2007; 52:965.

Kruger E, Heller DS: Adnexal torsion: a clinicopathologic review of 31 cases. J Reprod Med 1999; 44:71.

Kurjak A, Schulman H, Sosic A, et al: Transvaginal ultrasound, color flow, and Doppler waveform of the postmenopausal adnexal mass. Obstet Gynecol 1992; 80:917.

Kwa M et al The Intestinal Microbiome and Estrogen Receptor-Positive Female Breast Cancer J Natl Cancer Inst. 2016 Aug; 108(8): djw029

Leiserowitz GS. Managing ovarian masses during pregnancy. Obstet & Gynecol Survey. Jul 2006;61(7):463-70.

Li YM, Song LZ, Wang P, Jiang HJ.Observation on therapeutic effect of warming acupuncture and moxibustion combined with Chinese drugs on ovarian cysts Zhongguo Zhen Jiu. 2005 Aug;25(8):537-8. Shandong Provincial Institute of TCM, Jinan, China.

Lian F. TCM treatment of luteal phase defect--an analysis of 60 cases. J Tradit Chin Med. 1991 Jun;11(2):115-20.

Liepa GU, Sengupta A, Karsies D.Polycystic ovary syndrome (PCOS) and other androgen excess-related conditions: can changes in dietary intake make a difference? Nutr Clin Pract. 2008 Feb;23(1):63-71.

Ling FW, Slocumb JC. Use of trigger point injections in chronic pelvic pain. Obstet Gynecol Clin North Am 1993;20:809-15.

Mahdavi A, Berker B, Nezhat C, Nezhat F, Nezhat C. Laparoscopic management of ovarian cysts. Obstet Gynecol Clin North Am. Sep 2004;31(3):581-92, ix.

Marinov B, Tsachev K, Doganov N, Dzherov L, Markova M, Atanasova B, Shtereva K, Dimitrov R.Akush The zinc concentration of the blood serum in women with ovarian tumors Ginekol (Sofiia). 1998;37(4):16-8.

McDonald JM, Modesitt SC. The incidental postmenopausal adnexal mass. Clin Obstet & Gynecol. Sep 2006;49(3):506-16.

Milling LS. Is high hypnotic suggestibility necessary for successful hypnotic pain intervention? Curr Pain Headache Rep. 2008 Apr;12(2):98-102.

Modesitt SC, et al. (2003). Risk of malignancy in unilocular ovarian cystic tumors less than 10 centimeters in diameter. Obstetrics and Gynecology, 102(3): 594–599.

Mohammed HO, White ME, Guard CL, Smith MC, Mechor GD, Booker CW, Warnick LD, Dascanio JJ, Kenney DG. A case-control study of the association between blood selenium and cystic ovaries in lactating dairy cattle. J Dairy Sci. 1991 Jul;74(7):2180-5.

Montz FJ, Schlaerth JB, Morrow CP: The natural history of theca lutein cysts. Obstet Gynecol 1988; 72:247.

Mutter GL: Teratoma genetics and stem cells: A review. Obstet Gynecol Surv 1987; 42:661.

Norman RJ, Homan G, Moran L, Noakes M. Lifestyle choices, diet, and insulin sensitizers in polycystic ovary syndrome. Endocrine. 2006 Aug;30(1):35-43

Oltmann SC, Garcia N, Barber R, et al. Can we preoperatively risk stratify ovarian masses for malignancy? J Pediatr Surg 2010; 45:130.

Outwater EK, Siegelman ES, Talerman A, Dunton C: Ovarian fibromas and cystadenofibromas: MRI features of the fibrous component. J Magn Reson Imaging 1997; 7:465.

Parazzini F, Moroni S, Negri E, La Vecchia C, Dal Pino D, Ricci E. Risk factors for functional ovarian cysts. Epidemiology. Sep 1996;7(5):547-9.

Parker MF, Conslato SS, Chang AS, et al: Chemical analysis of adnexal cyst fluid. Gynecol Oncol 1999; 73:16.

Peters WA, Thiagarajah S, Thornton WN: Ovarian hemorrhage in patients receiving anticoagulant therapy. J Reprod Med 1979; 22:82.

Pham T, Scofield RH. 13-cis-Retinoic acid (isotretinoin) unmasking of clinical polycystic ovary syndrome. Endocr Pract. 2007 Nov-Dec;13(7):776-9.

Raziel A, Ron-El R, Pansky M, et al: Current management of ruptured corpus luteum. Eur J Obstet Gynecol Reprod Biol 1993; 50:77.

Russell AL, McCarty MF. DL-phenylalanine markedly potentiates opiate analgesia - an example of nutrient/pharmaceutical up-regulation of the endogenous analgesia system. Med Hypotheses. 2000 Oct;55(4):283-8.

Schmeler KM, Mayo-Smith WW, Peipert JF, et al. Adnexal masses in pregnancy: surgery compared with observation. Obstet Gynecol. May 2005;105(5 Pt 1):1098-103.

Setji TL, Brown AJ. Polycystic ovary syndrome: diagnosis and treatment. Am J Med. Feb 2007;120(2):128-32.

Song JJ, Yan ME, Wu XK, Hou LH. Progress of integrative Chinese and Western medicine in treating polycystic ovarian syndrome caused infertility. Gynecological and Obstetric Department, First Hospital, Heilongjiang University of Traditional Chinese Medicine, Harbin (150040). Chin J Integr Med. 2006 Dec;12(4):312-6.

Song YN, Zhu L, Lang JH. Recurrent mature ovarian teratomas: retrospective analysis of 20 cases Department of Obstetrics and Gynecology, Peking Union Medical College Hospital, Peking Union Medical College, Chinese Academy of Medical Science, Beijing 100730, China. Zhonghua Yi Xue Za Zhi. 2007 May 8;87(17):1184-6.

Stein AL, Koonings PP, Schlaerth JB, et al: Relative frequency of malignant parovarian tumors: Should parovarian tumors be aspirated?. Obstet Gynecol 1990; 75:1029.

Steinkampf MP, Hammond KR, Blackwell RE. Hormonal treatment of functional ovarian cysts: a randomized, prospective study. Fertil Steril. Nov 1990;54(5):775-7.

Survey and health assessment of chemicals substances in sex toys: http://www2.mst.dk/common/Udgivramme/Frame.asp?pg=http://www2.mst.dk/udgiv/publications/2006/87-7052-227-8/html/helepubl_eng.htm

Thys-Jacobs S, Donovan D, Papadopoulos A, Sarrel P, Bilezikian JP.

Tsai HJ. Suitable timing of surgical intervention for ruptured ovarian endometrioma. Taiwan J Obstet Gynecol 2015; 54:105.

Ushiroyama T, Ikeda A, Higashio S, Hosotani T, Yamashita H, Yamashita Y, Suzuki Y, Ueki M.J Unkei-to for correcting luteal phase defects. Reprod Med. 2003 Sep;48(9):729-34.

Vitamin D and calcium dysregulation in the polycystic ovarian syndrome. Steroids. 1999 Jun;64(6):430-5.

Wickenheisser JK, Nelson-DeGrave VL, Hendricks KL, Legro RS, Strauss JF 3rd, McAllister JM. Retinoids and retinol differentially regulate steroid biosynthesis in ovarian theca cells isolated from normal cycling women and women with polycystic ovary syndrome. J Clin Endocrinol Metab. 2005 Aug;90(8):4858-65.

World Gastroenterology Organisation. Probiotics and prebiotics 2017. https://www.worldgastroenterology.org/UserFiles/file/guidelines/probiotics-and-prebiotics-english-2017.pdf

Zhang HY, Yu XZ, Wang GL. Preliminary report of the treatment of luteal phase defect by replenishing kidney. An analysis of 53 cases[Article in Chinese] Zhongguo Zhong Xi Yi Jie He Za Zhi. 1992 Aug;12(8):473-4, 452-3.

Zhao X, Liu JL, Chen SR, Liu Y. Analysis of relative factors influencing recurrence of endometriosis after operation treatment Department of Obstetrics and Gynecology, the Affiliated Hospital of Zunyi Medical College, Zunyi 563003, China. Zhonghua Fu Chan Ke Za Zhi. 2006 Oct;41(10):669-71.

About The Author

Quadruple board certified in Obstetrics & Gynecology, Gynecologic Oncology, and Integrative & Holistic Medicine (two boards), Dr. Steven Vasilev MD, MBA, FACOG, FACS, FACN, ABIHM, ABOIM is a nationally recognized cancer surgeon who specializes in advanced minimally invasive robotic surgery. Dr. Vasilev strongly supports patient-centered integrative oncology care as the 21st-century new gold standard. Given that the word doctor derives from the word docere, he firmly believes the most skilled doctor must also be a patient teacher and caring guide.

Dr. Vasilev is also a nationally known educator and clinical researcher. He has served as faculty at multiple medical schools and cancer centers including UCLA, USC, UC Irvine, and the City of Hope. He is currently a Professor at Loma Linda University School of Medicine and John Wayne Cancer Institute in Santa Monica, California. He has trained over two hundred fifty doctors in complex surgery and integrative cancer care. As an innovative master surgeon, he performs 95% of his surgeries using advanced minimally invasive laparoscopy and high-tech robotics.

As an author, he has published and contributed to hundreds of articles, research meeting abstracts, and book chapters. He also authored a textbook on the topic of scientific evidence based perioperative and supportive care as well as a book on holistic integrative cancer care.

Among many awards, Best Doctors® has listed him among the nation's top 5% of doctors for nineteen years running.

As a physician who also holds an MBA degree from the prestigious UCLA Anderson School, Dr. Vasilev has a keen sense of science-supported truth vs. marketing hyperbole. So, in practice and in this book, he shares how to find the best evidence supported natural support options. At the same time, he strives to keep your "B.S.-meter" tuned up to help you avoid useless and harmful treatments. As a true certified multidimensional and authoritative expert in both Western and Eastern natural approaches to women's healthcare, he forges an integrative path for the reader to follow towards healthy thriving and ovarian cyst prevention.

www.ingramcontent.com/pod-product-compliance
Lightning Source LLC
Chambersburg PA
CBHW022122280326
41933CB00007B/511
9781942065272